THE METABOLISM MAKEOVER
WORKBOOK

MEGAN HANSEN, RDN

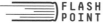
FLASH POINT

This book is dedicated to the Metabolism Makeover community, who enthusiastically allow me to test my methods and madness before bringing them to the world.

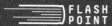

Published by Flashpoint™ Books, Seattle
www.flashpointbooks.com

Produced by Girl Friday Productions

Design: Rachel Marek
Production editorial: Reshma Kooner
Project management: Emilie Sandoz-Voyer

Image credits: cover and interior, © Emily Hart | Mood + Theory (author photo) and Tim Robbins (icon pattern); vi–ix, xi, 2, 3, 7, 13, 19, 23, 26, 29, 36, 108, 110, 123, 172 (handdrawn elements) by Shutterstock users ebi_ko, Martyshova Maria, and Polina Tomtosova.

ISBN (paperback): 978-1-959411-60-4

First edition

CONTENTS

The Way We're Wired

I know you—because I've been you. You've been dieting as long as you can remember, and you're sick and tired of the amount of space food—and your weight—takes up in your brain. You can't even imagine what it would be like to not think about lunch while you're eating breakfast, or dinner while you're eating lunch. You would give *anything* to never start over on yet another Monday, but you don't even know where to start to make that a reality. And quite frankly, you're tired of your own bullshit. Sure, you've got some legitimate excuses for why this diet failed or why that exercise program didn't work, but for the most part, you blame yourself for being where you are. You're frustrated, and you just want to feel better in your body and about your body.

Here are some things that might be holding you back:

> » *I can do a million hard things, but I always fail at* this. *No matter what I do, it doesn't work.*

> » *I am confused by all the different diets, fads, and right-versus-wrong mentality.*

> » *I lack the motivation to change. What's wrong with me?*

> » *I'm great at getting started, but I am not consistent.*

> » *I want to see real change in my body, but at this point, I don't know how.*

Not only have I had the same struggles as you, but I've also worked with thousands of clients in the same boat. Here's a list of common experiences. Check the ones that resonate with you.

☐ Do you have frequent cravings?

☐ Are you addicted to sugar?

☐ Are you always hungry?

☐ Are you never hungry for breakfast?

☐ Do you get hangry?

☐ Do you need to eat every two to three hours?

☐ Do you experience afternoon energy crashes?

☐ Do you have PCOS, irregular periods, or painful periods?

☐ Do you feel like you do everything right but can't lose weight?

☐ Are you good all week but go overboard on the weekends?

☐ Do you know what to do to lose weight, but you just can't seem to make yourself do it?

If you answered yes to any of these questions, whether one or all eleven, you are exactly like 100 percent of the women I work with, and you are most certainly **in the right place**.

In order to make **real changes** *happen, we need to know* **how our bodies work.**

This workbook is an actionable companion to my book *Metabolism Makeover: Ditch the Diet, Train Your Brain, Drop the Weight for Good.* The biggest takeaway I learned throughout my own weight loss journey is that knowledge is critical. In order to make real changes happen, we need to know how our bodies work, which is why I wrote *Metabolism Makeover.* That book is a great place to start over with your relationship to eating and weight loss. I like to think of it as the owner's manual for your body that you were never given.

But as G.I. Joe has been known to say, "Knowing is only half the battle." Losing weight and keeping it off involves a heck of a lot more than just diet and exercise. We need to apply that knowing to three areas:

1. Increasing self-awareness to become conscious of our choices
2. Installing new habits and shifting beliefs that are keeping us stuck
3. Focusing our attention on the person we know we can become

And much of this has to do with how our brains are wired. There is a conscious part of our brain, the part of our thinking, feeling, and actions that we are fully aware of, and the subconscious part, which is where our deeper mental processes take place without us really knowing what's going on in there. The way we think about ourselves, our identities, and our belief systems is embedded in our subconscious mind, and we consistently make unconscious decisions based on those identities and beliefs.

Changing your diet and going to the gym is a decision you make with your conscious mind, and the conscious mind primarily relies on willpower. If you're like me, willpower lasts only as long as you're feeling excited about a change and have the energy for it. But when willpower runs out, that's where the subconscious takes over, and this part of your mind is hardwired to make the best decisions it can with the information it has. Sticking to new habits becomes difficult when you have another goal (for instance, indulging in a true-crime docuseries marathon) that conflicts with your new intentions (getting eight hours of sleep).

Your conscious mind excels at coming up with rationalizations to stick to the status quo, and willpower cannot override the subconscious when it's found a better reason to stay up late than go to bed. This means that if your subconscious mind isn't on board with your habits, you'll go right back to what's "comfortable," like skipping the gym and ordering takeout.

I know it feels like you're consciously in charge of all the choices you make, but the truth is that 95 percent of our daily decisions are made from our subconscious—from our in-grained patterns, beliefs, and understandings of the world. While that's super useful when you automatically brake to not hit a squirrel while driving, it's less useful when you're try-ing to lose weight. This is why every time you've gone on a diet, it "works" until it doesn't anymore. You need this part of the mind to get on board with your new habits.

The truth is that (95%) *of our daily decisions are made from our subconscious.*

The exercises and tools in this workbook are designed to do exactly that: revamp your subconscious mind so it can get with the program and work with your conscious goals instead of against them. Once your subconscious gets on board, behavior and decisions follow.

WHAT TO EXPECT

You might be thinking, *Where do I start?* The answer? Right here! This workbook will guide you through a one-year mindset and metabolism makeover. After working with over eight thousand clients, I know the key ingredients required for lasting results. This workbook is a carbon copy of the path my most successful clients take.

Most weight loss workbooks offer instruction for 4 to 8 weeks. This one is 52. Why? TikTok might promise you that the latest weight loss hack will have you losing 10 pounds overnight, but I don't think you're interested in losing weight just to gain it all back. I think you're here because you want something with staying power. This time around, you've made a choice to really commit to yourself.

We begin with a four-week commitment that's easy to say yes to. This is designed to give you some quick results and momentum—because we're human and we love that dopamine hit! But it will also offer the path to staying power and long-term results.

Before I ask you to commit to even the first four weeks, let me be clear on how the metabolism makeover approach is different from what you've tried before:

Traditional approach to weight loss	Metabolism makeover framework
Partial view of what it takes to lose weight: diet and exercise	360-degree view of what it takes to lose weight: blood sugar control, muscle, movement, sleep, stress management, and gut health
Decrease calories	Increase metabolism
Burn calories	Build muscle
Work out harder	Work out smarter
Track your food	Tune in to internal calorie counters: your hunger and satiety hormones
Weight loss ✗	Fat loss ✓
Macro habits: overhaul your diet, clean out your pantry, gym 5 days a week, meal prep every meal	Micro habits: 30 grams of protein at breakfast, prep 2 proteins a week, 20-minute power walks, laying out workout clothes before bed
~~Eat this, not that~~	Understanding how your body's metabolism works, and having the freedom to choose what foods you love to eat based on that knowledge
Lose 10 pounds in 10 days	Lose fat and gain sexy, lean muscle for life
Follow a plan like a robot, until you fall off the wagon	Gain enough self-awareness around your habits that they become easy to integrate into your life
Use willpower to muscle through habit change	Hack the subconscious mind to put your habits on autopilot—no willpower required
Assumes life never throws you a curveball—date night, sick kids, three soccer games this week, forgetting to make dinner, weekends, a catered lunch	Creates awareness through a weekly preview and review process, as well as tools to support you in the moment when shit hits the fan
The only strategy offered is behavior change	The strategy is learning how your body's metabolism works so decisions can be made on autopilot instead of using willpower

You have the power to change your body. But it doesn't stop there. I've had the honor of witnessing people from all age ranges and backgrounds repair their metabolism, lose weight, and heal their relationship with food. And here's what I can tell you about them: those who made the decision to ditch the diet industry's rules quite literally changed their entire lives.

HOW TO USE THIS WORKBOOK

The workbook is separated into four parts.

Part One: Here's How Your Body Works

We start at the beginning, with an understanding of how your body actually works. I'll teach you the key concepts about fat loss and your body's metabolism. This knowledge is an essential step to greater self-awareness and harnessing your subconscious to make decisions that support your vision. I'm really offering only a crash course in this workbook, but you can check out *Metabolism Makeover* for a more comprehensive look at the inner workings of the body.

Part Two: Who Are You?

In the past, you've likely made the mistake of jumping right in to achieve your goal. While this seems like the right path to take, I explain in this section why this hasn't worked out in the long run. Instead, creating a vision for YOU (that's the big, juicy, empowered version of yourself you know is in there) is a key part of this process. Once you craft a vision and choose a destination for yourself, you'll know exactly where you're going. Then, you can easily map your journey and never end up where you *don't* want to be ever again. In this part, you'll also define your why—a powerful exercise that blows clients away time and again. We will also address any of those limiting beliefs that are pumping the brakes on your goals.

Part Three: Your Four-Week Jump Start

With a firm foundation in the why, we'll now jump into the how. Although long-term, sustainable fat loss requires far more than four weeks, in this part, I'll help you create some quick wins with the four most effective micro habits my clients implement. Focusing on just these four steps gives you some immediate momentum as well as some space to take your new vision and reprogrammed subconscious beliefs out for a test drive. The stakes are low here, so it's a time to play around and see what works for you.

Part Four: Your Road Map for the Rest of the Year

After you complete your first four weeks, we'll celebrate your wins, look at what worked and what didn't, and address some common questions clients have when facing the rest of their year. From there, you will be in the driver's seat to design the next 48 weeks in a sustainable and (dare I say) fun way that will lead you to your YOU. This year is the gateway to the rest of your life as the YOU that you've always imagined. But don't worry—I will give you all the tools you need to make this happen.

This workbook is not just another set of strict rules to follow. It's not another get-thin-quick scheme or fad diet plan. Instead, it's a science-backed road map that will empower you to make decisions about what to eat, how to move, and how to live in a way that supports your body, no matter what season of life you are in.

Let's get started!
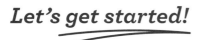

PART ONE

Here's How Your Body Works

We need to eat to live, and the calories from food sources like protein, fiber, and carbs give us the energy to keep the machine that is our body running smoothly. Metabolism is the process where your body takes those calories and turns them into energy. It dictates how your body breaks down and utilizes everything you put into your mouth.

The number of calories burned each day carrying out basic functions (things like breathing, pumping blood, regulating hormone levels, and repairing cells) is your basal metabolic rate (BMR). So while it's important to move and exercise to burn calories, the majority of the calories you burn each day is through your BMR. When your metabolism is functioning optimally, you will burn more calories at rest, which is why optimizing your metabolism over simply focusing on calories is key.

The key takeaway here is that metabolism is really just another way of saying how the body utilizes the calories you consume. So how can you make sure your metabolism is utilizing all of its calories instead of storing them as fat? To answer this question, we have to look at the six pillars of what I call the Metabolic Ecosystem.

THE METABOLIC ECOSYSTEM

There are six pillars that create the foundation of your metabolic health:

1. *Blood sugar control*
2. *Muscle*
3. *Movement*
4. *Good sleep*
5. *Stress management*
6. *A healthy gut*

Understanding and regaining control over these pillars is your golden ticket not just for losing weight but for keeping it off for good.

Importantly, these pillars are not independent variables. This is an interconnected system, and if one pillar is being neglected, it can have a domino effect on the entire ecosystem. If this sounds like a lot to juggle already, don't panic! This system is empowering, not limiting. Once you have an understanding of each pillar, you will have so many more opportunities to fire up your metabolism and take care of your body outside of just diet and exercise.

We'll take a brief look at all the pillars and the most important facts to know about each. There are also some reflection questions and activities throughout this section, so grab a pen!

*Metabolism is really just another way of saying **how the body utilizes the calories you consume**.*

Pillar #1: Blood Sugar Control

Blood sugar is the amount of glucose (sugar) in the blood. It is our body's primary source of energy. When we eat carbohydrates, our blood sugar rises, the pancreas releases insulin, and the insulin scoops up the glucose and delivers it to our cells, which then turn the glucose into energy.

The problem is that when glucose rises too quickly—like after a carb-heavy bowl of pasta, a sugary caramel macchiato, or even a banana on an empty stomach—there is a subsequent crash that signals to the brain that the body needs more sugar. These blood sugar spikes and dips lead to energy crashes, cravings, increased hunger, and the shutdown of fat-burning mechanisms. On the other hand, when blood sugar levels are steady, the body is able to burn fat.

Eating protein, healthy fat, and fiber—what I call PHFF—alongside carbohydrates will generally maintain steady blood sugar levels and prevent spikes and crashes. When you master controlling blood sugar, you'll have more energy and fewer cravings, feel more in control around food, and unlock your body's internal fat-burning mechanisms.

What You Need to Know

1. The main signs of **dysregulated blood sugar** are getting hangry, experiencing energy crashes, not being able to go at least four hours between meals, getting cravings, having brain fog, and feeling irritable.

2. **Chronically elevated blood sugar** leads to weight loss resistance, hormone imbalances, insulin resistance, and type 2 diabetes.

3. **Protein is the most satiating macronutrient.** Eating protein at every meal will ensure you're staying full while losing weight. Shoot for at least 30 grams of protein per meal from sources like eggs, responsibly sourced animal meats and seafood, dairy, beans, lentils, nuts, tofu, and seeds.

4. **Healthy fats are a powerful blood sugar modulator.** Eating fat with carbs will slow the blood sugar response. A serving of fat is about 10 grams, and most women need at least 60 grams of fat per day for healthy hormones. This can look like anywhere from one to three servings of fat per meal. Healthy fats include nuts, seeds, avocados, olive oil, and butter.

5. **Fiber is similar to fat in its blood-sugar-controlling properties, and it also turns off hunger hormones.** I recommend at least 25 grams of fiber per day for optimal blood sugar control and appetite regulation. Fiber can be found in nonstarchy vegetables like broccoli, cauliflower, and asparagus, as well as in berries, apples, chia seeds, beans, lentils, nuts, and grains.

6. **Keep starchy carbs** like rice, quinoa, beans, pasta, potatoes, tortillas, couscous, and bread **to 30–40 grams of carbs per meal** to keep blood sugar under control. (This does not include carbs from dairy, vegetables, fruit, nuts, and seeds.)

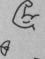

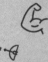
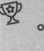

Activity: Get to Know Your Food

Open up your pantry and look at your food labels to get an idea of what a serving **(30–40 grams) of starchy carbs** looks like.

rice _____	corn _____
pasta _____	tortillas _____
lentil pasta _____	_____
quinoa _____	_____
bread _____	_____
potatoes _____	_____

Now look at your food labels to get an idea of what a serving **(~10 grams) of fat** looks like.

peanut butter _____	cheddar cheese _____
olives _____	almonds _____
butter _____	_____
olive oil _____	_____
guacamole _____	_____
coconut milk (canned) _____	_____

Check your labels and look at **how much protein** is in some of your most common foods.

4 oz chicken breast _____	protein powder _____
1 can of tuna _____	beans _____
4 oz ground beef _____	peanut butter _____
½ cup cottage cheese _____	_____
½ cup plain Greek yogurt _____	_____
beef stick / beef jerky _____	_____
mozzarella cheese _____	_____

Reflection Questions

What patterns do you notice around your energy throughout the day?

What kinds of cravings do you have, and how do you deal with them?

How long can you typically go between meals before you start to feel hunger?

Reflect on your meals from a few recent days. Did they follow the PHFF guidelines? Based on what you just learned about blood sugar control, how did those food choices impact your blood sugar? What could you have done differently?

Pillar #2: Muscle

The reasons to build muscle are endless, but when it comes to changing your body, muscle has two main perks: (1) it looks great in a tank top and (2) the more you have, the more calories you burn.

Muscle is calorically expensive, meaning the body has to burn a lot of calories just to keep it. More muscle increases your BMR, which makes up 55–70 percent of your daily calorie burn. Build more muscle, burn more calories (in your sleep!). You can build and maintain muscle two ways. The first is through strength training, which means exercising your muscles under tension. The second way to build and maintain muscle is through eating enough protein to activate muscle protein synthesis.

Build more muscle, burn more calories (in your sleep!).

What You Need to Know

1. As a woman, **building muscle does not mean you will get bulky** unless you are taking hormones. "Getting big" requires a lot of testosterone.

2. **Effective ways to strength train** include lifting weights, using resistance bands, or even just using your own body weight.

3. **Eating at least 30 grams of animal protein in a meal** generally triggers muscle protein synthesis. Do this three times a day and you'll be in good shape for triggering muscle growth.

4. If you consume no or limited animal products, it will be difficult to trigger muscle protein synthesis because you will fall short on the amino acids it takes to do so. A way around this is to **find a plant-based protein powder with added amino acids** and make a shake for breakfast. These are often classified as "sports" protein powders that are designed with your muscles in mind. Another option is to take an essential amino acid supplement. You can find recommendations for both in the resource section.

5. No matter the technique you choose, your **strength training should be based around the idea of *progressive overload***, which means continually increasing your reps or weight. For example, if you do 20 push-ups one training day, the next time, do 21. Or, if you did 10 bicep curls at 10 pounds one week, do 11 reps the next week or try 12.5–pound dumbbells.

6. A great way to never see progress at the gym is by spending every day at the gym. **Your muscles need time to recover or they'll never build.** Take at least two rest days per week.

7. **Long, high-intensity workouts** like boot camps, spin classes, and six-mile runs may burn a lot of calories, but doing these types of workouts every day while in a calorie deficit will eventually lead the body to becoming more efficient at burning those calories. So while your Apple Watch may say you burned 600 calories, you may have burned only 100.

8. While any exercise is better than no exercise, barre, Pilates, yoga, and other classes that focus only on accessory muscles do not lead to burning fat. **While cardio-focused workouts do burn fat, they also have a tendency to burn muscle when done regularly**, and they don't always help you keep weight off in the long term.

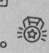
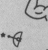

Activity: Three-Day Strength Routine

Here is a basic three-day strength routine to get you started. If you are new to weights, I encourage you to go to metabolismmakeover.co/resources to find videos of each exercise. You will also find a no-equipment workout program. You can give these a shot at a local gym or pick up some dumbbells to try at home. In the resource section in the back of this workbook, I include some additional workout programs that you may want to try as well. A great way to see and amplify your progress is to track your weights and reps. This way, you can slowly increase in weights or reps each week—a little more weight or one more rep. Your notes app on your phone works great, though there is some space right in this workbook to get you started.

	EXERCISE	SETS	REPS
DAY 1	Split squats	2	8–12
	Bent-over rows	3	8–12
	Bench press	3	8–12
	Romanian dead lift	4	8–12
	Push-ups	3	10–15
	Bicep curls	3	10–15
DAY 2	Bench step-ups	2	12–15
	Glute bridge	2	12–15
	Sissy squats	2	8–15
	Leaning lateral raise	3	10–15
	Banded lateral raise	3	10–15
	Overhead triceps extension	2	10–15
DAY 3	Front squats	2	12–15
	Overhead press	3	8–12
	Chest flies	2	12–15
	One-arm bent-over rows	2	10–12 per arm
	Upright rows	2	10–15
	V-ups	1 minute	
	Reverse crunches	1 minute	

EXERCISE	SETS	REPS	WEIGHT

Check out the Metabolism Makeover resources page for exercise videos, printable charts, and more.

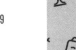

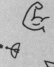

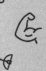

Reflection Questions

What barriers to strength training do you experience? Is it time, lack of access to a gym, an injury? What can you do to address those barriers?

_____

_____

_____

_____

_____

_____

_____

Think about your current weekly workout routine. What changes can you make to prioritize building muscle?

_____

_____

_____

_____

_____

_____

_____

When you think about working out, what is your focus? Burning calories? Getting stronger?

_____

_____

_____

_____

_____

_____

A great way to never **see progress at the gym** *is by spending every day at the gym. Your muscles need time to recover or they'll never build.* **Take at least two rest days per week.**

Pillar #3: Movement

If you hit the gym for 1 hour five to six times per week, then get your groceries and meals delivered while sitting at your desk or lying on the couch or bed for the remaining 23 hours, you fall into the category of *actively sedentary*, which can lead to sickness, weight gain, and mobility issues later in life. Yikes!

Movement is key to a healthy body and weight, especially as you age. I define movement as *living in motion*. It's any low-impact physical activity, such as walking, housework, gardening, hiking, squatting down to pick up a toddler or heavy box, and standing instead of sitting at your desk. Aside from a sedentary lifestyle contributing to a whole litany of health complications, movement is vital when it comes to metabolic flexibility, blood sugar control, stress relief, and the ability to maintain movement as we age. Along with all those benefits, the more you move, the more calories you burn.

Movement is key to a healthy body and weight, especially as you age.

What You Need to Know

1. Zone 2 cardio, or as I like to call it, *power walking*, is **one of the most efficient ways to increase metabolic flexibility**, meaning the body's metabolism is adaptable enough to use whatever fuel is available to it. The body can then easily burn fat for energy instead of always relying on carbohydrates. Zone 2 cardio is characterized by being able to maintain a conversation but having to pause on occasion to take a breath.

2. Most experts agree that **150–180 minutes per week of zone 2 cardio** is important for metabolic and longevity benefits.

3. The second-most effective way to control blood sugar outside of diet is moving your body after meals. A 20-minute walk or bike ride after a meal can reduce blood sugar levels. **Steady blood sugar = less insulin = more fat burned.**

4. No one has time to add one more thing to their day. **Add movement to the activities you already do every day** by standing or pacing during work calls, getting everyone outside for family activities, holding yoga poses while watching TV, or sneaking in random movement, like doing calf raises while brushing your teeth.

5. You can also **"habit stack" movement with other pillars of the Metabolic Ecosystem**: take a walk in the morning sunlight to help you sleep better, add a podcast or call a friend while walking for stress relief, or walk after meals to stabilize blood sugar.

6. **Have fun with movement** by getting on the playground, pulling out your old bike, and getting down on the ground to play with your kids or dog.

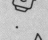

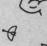
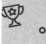

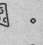
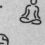

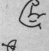

Activity: Track Your Day in Detail

Pick a day where you can keep this workbook beside you to detail your entire day every 30 minutes. At the end of your day, look through the list and make notes of where you can add in more movement.

TIME	WHAT I'M DOING	CAN I ADD MOVEMENT?
5:00 a.m.		
5:30 a.m.		
6:00 a.m.		
6:30 a.m.		
7:00 a.m.		
7:30 a.m.		
8:00 a.m.		
8:30 a.m.		
9:00 a.m.		
9:30 a.m.		
10:00 a.m.		
10:30 a.m.		
11:00 a.m.		
11:30 a.m.		
12:00 p.m.		
12:30 p.m.		
1:00 p.m.		
1:30 p.m.		
2:00 p.m.		
2:30 p.m.		
3:00 p.m.		
3:30 p.m.		
4:00 p.m.		

TIME	WHAT I'M DOING	CAN I ADD MOVEMENT?
4:30 p.m.		
5:00 p.m.		
5:30 p.m.		
6:00 p.m.		
6:30 p.m.		
7:00 p.m.		
7:30 p.m.		
8:00 p.m.		
8:30 p.m.		
9:00 p.m.		
9:30 p.m.		
10:00 p.m.		
10:30 p.m.		
11:00 p.m.		
11:30 p.m.		
12:00 a.m.		
12:30 a.m.		
1:00 a.m.		
1:30 a.m.		
2:00 a.m.		
2:30 a.m.		
3:00 a.m.		
3:30 a.m.		
4:00 a.m.		
4:30 a.m.		

Notes:

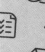
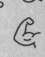
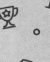

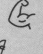

Reflection Questions

Think about things that are a part of your daily or weekly routine such as watching TV, doing chores, and listening to podcasts. What are some easy movements you can add to these tasks?

_____

_____

_____

_____

_____

_____

_____

_____

_____

What are some creative ways you can move your body more, aside from going for a walk?

_____

_____

_____

_____

_____

_____

_____

_____

If you currently struggle to get in movement, what are your biggest barriers? What can you do to address those barriers?

_____

_____

_____

_____

_____

_____

_____

_____

No one has time to add one more thing to their day. **Add movement to the activities you already do** *every day.*

Pillar #4: Good Sleep

You know sleep is important, but you may not know how important sleep is when it comes to hunger, satiety, cravings, and metabolism. Sleep is when we renew and regenerate our system. Tissues are repaired, cells detox and turn over, and hormones—including hormones that regulate our appetite and weight—are produced and regulated.

Getting less than 6 hours of sleep while losing weight results in 55 percent *less* fat loss and 60 percent *more* muscle loss than getting 8.5 hours of sleep. It also increases the hunger hormone (ghrelin) and decreases the satiety hormone (leptin), leading you to seek out highly craveable (read: sugary and carb-dense) foods and consume an average of 270 more calories per day. TL;DR: good things happen when you get more sleep.

Good things happen *when you get more sleep.*

What You Need to Know

1. The American Academy of Sleep Medicine recommends getting between **seven and nine hours of sleep per night**.

2. **Your sleep cycle, regulated by your circadian rhythm, is largely impacted by light.** Getting outside within a few hours of sunrise begins a chemical reaction in the body that releases melatonin at the appropriate time in the evening. This works only if you are looking (safely) in the direction of the sun for 10 minutes on a sunny day or 30 minutes on a cloudy day.

3. Turning down the lights, taking a walk at sunset, and avoiding screens or wearing blue-light blockers in the evening all signal to the body that it's nighttime, thus **preparing the body for an easy transition to sleep**.

4. **Alcohol disrupts REM sleep** and causes variable blood sugar levels that can wake you up in the night or at the very least cause restless sleep. Even just one drink! Where possible, cut out drinking at least during the week.

5. **Avoid caffeine 8 to 10 hours before bedtime**—yes, this basically means coffee in the morning only. To start scaling back, have your last cup 15 minutes earlier each day until you settle on a time that doesn't seem to affect sleep.

6. **Prioritize consistency as much as possible.** Even if you're working the night shift only four days per week, stay as close to your night shift sleeping and eating schedule as you can.

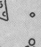

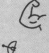

Activity: Set a Bedtime Routine

A big reason we don't get enough sleep or we experience disruptive sleep is because we aren't preparing our bodies and minds for bed effectively. To set yourself up for successful sleep each night, set a minimal bedtime routine. If you have kids, you know what this is. It's a series of nonnegotiable steps that you take every night, no matter what, to trigger the brain to be ready for sleep. You can always add to this routine, but the point is to keep it simple so you can do it every day—no matter where you're laying down your head. There are infinite ways to go about this, but here are a few examples:

- ☐ Turn down unnecessary lights around the house, and put on blue-light blockers after dinner.
- ☐ Put your phone away at 8:00 p.m.
- ☐ Take an Epsom salt bath or hot shower.
- ☐ Be in bed by 9:00 p.m. and read (not on a screen!) until you fall asleep.

Write out a minimal bedtime routine for yourself and stick to it for at least a week. Then, feel free to make changes or additions as needed.

_____
_____
_____
_____
_____
_____
_____
_____
_____
_____
_____

Reflection Questions

How many hours of sleep are you currently getting on average? If less than seven hours, what can you do, beginning today, to increase that?

What patterns in your cravings and hunger levels have you noticed on days you sleep less?

What do you believe your biggest barriers are to getting adequate sleep? How can you address those barriers?

Pillar #5: Stress Management

Stress can be classified as anything that taxes the body or mind, and aside from the obvious reasons we like to avoid it, stress has a massive impact on metabolic health. Our diet, exercise regimen, sleep habits, gut health, and mindset all contribute to our body's daily stress load.

Importantly, while your mind perceives different stressors in different ways, your body does not. The body recognizes physical stressors in the same category as mental and emotional stressors. So whether you're doing a sweaty spin class or having an argument, your brain receives the signal about stress the same way: releasing adrenaline and then cortisol to increase your heart rate, sharpen your focus, and energize your body for action. This is a natural and useful response; the issue comes when the body is constantly experiencing stress, what is called *chronic stress*.

When the body is in a state of chronic stress, adrenaline and cortisol remain elevated, causing damage to blood vessels, an increased risk of heart attack and stroke, high blood sugar levels, insulin resistance, hormonal imbalances, an increase in belly fat, gut microbiome dysfunction, and increased cravings.

In my practice, stress is the number one cause of weight loss resistance. This includes overexercising, undereating, physiological stress like marital or financial stress, and internal stress like chronic disease or autoimmune disease.

While your **mind** *perceives different stressors in different ways,* **your body does not**.

What You Need to Know

Stress comes in two forms: physiological and psychological. Both of these categories include stressors that are both in and out of our control. We can remove controllable stressors and learn to increase our capacity for life's inevitable uncontrollable stressors.

Physiological

- getting less than 7 hours of sleep
- low-carb diets
- high-intensity workouts more than twice per week
- marathon training
- undereating
- no rest days
- fasted workouts
- 16+ hours of intermittent fasting
- too much caffeine
- blood sugar swings
- leaky gut

Psychological

- lack of boundaries
- fixation with being busy
- negative self-talk
- watching the news
- phone notifications
- worrying about things that haven't happened
- sweating the small stuff
- toxic friends
- a shitty romantic partner
- doomscrolling

Keeping a regular nervous system practice is essential for keeping stress levels under control. Here is an inexhaustive list of some powerful techniques to increase your daily capacity for stress:

- doing breath work
- grounding
- getting into nature
- walking
- taking Epsom salt baths
- cuddling or a 30-second hug

- pausing and feeling into your body when anxiety strikes
- meditating
- doing yoga or tai chi
- resting without screens
- journaling

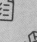

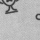

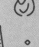

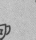

Activity: What Are Your Stressors?

Are you overstressed? Check off all the boxes that apply to you.

☐ At bedtime, I am tired but wired and struggle to fall asleep.

☐ I often have low energy.

☐ I sometimes feel I function best under stress.

☐ My menstrual cycle is inconsistent or nonexistent.

☐ I experience mood swings, like feeling irritable for no reason.

☐ I have brain fog or trouble focusing consistently.

☐ I have anxiety more days than not.

☐ I am prone to starting several projects at once or overcommitting.

If you checked more than one of the above, **you are likely overstressed**. Over time, this can have a significant, negative impact on your ability to lose weight.

Some stressors are just an unavoidable part of life. But we can have control over other stressors. What stressors are you experiencing that you can immediately remove from your life? Write out your most common stressors and decide which ones can be removed this week.

Stressors	Stressors I'm committing to removing
	☐
	☐
	☐
	☐
	☐
	☐
	☐
	☐
	☐
	☐
	☐
	☐

Activity: Grounding Practice

Practice this simple grounding technique every day for one week, then come back to answer the following reflection questions.

DAILY GROUNDING TECHNIQUE

When you first wake up in the morning, let your feet hit the floor and **pause**.

Close your eyes and feel into your feet. Imagine all of the energy in your body draining to the bottoms of your feet. Any thoughts, worries, or stress you might be experiencing upon waking is just going to go right into the ground.

Then, take a moment for gratitude. Choose at least three things to be thankful for and speak them out loud or in your head. If you like this practice, this is also a good time to repeat your YOU statements that you will craft in part 2 of this workbook (see page 52).

When you feel calm and grounded, stand up and go about your day.

COMPLETED DAILY GROUNDING TECHNIQUE ☑

Day 1	Day 2	Day 3	Day 4	Day 5	Day 6	Day 7
☐	☐	☐	☐	☐	☐	☐

Reflection Questions

How are you currently managing your stress? If you can't answer this question, what changes can you make this week?

_____

_____

_____

_____

_____

_____

What patterns do you notice on days you are particularly stressed, especially in terms of eating, exercise, and sleep?

_____

_____

_____

_____

_____

_____

_____

What did you notice after a week of doing the grounding practice? Were there any differences in how you felt as you began the day? What about the rest of the day?

_____

_____

_____

_____

_____

_____

Pillar #6: A Healthy Gut

I can't do justice to this complex topic in this workbook. My goal here is to give you some basic, foundational information and some easy steps to kick-start taking care of your gut at home.

Gut health refers to the function and balance of the bacteria that populate the gastrointestinal system, a.k.a. the GI tract or gut. These bacteria, also known as the *microbiome*, release chemicals as they interact with the foods we eat, and those chemicals regulate our immune system and metabolism, as well as communicate with our brain and organs. A healthy gut microbiome communicates with cells all over the body, from your nervous system to your immune system to your digestive system to your mental health—and to your metabolism.

An unhealthy gut triggers chronic inflammation, which can be a root cause of a variety of health issues and even an increased mortality rate. For our purposes, I'm focusing on the fact that it's one of the primary sources of weight loss resistance. This is mainly because when the body is focused on fighting inflammation, burning fat is deprioritized.

Minerals play several crucial roles in the body that include enzyme activity, hormone regulation, energy production, and helping shape the gut microbiome. When the body is low—or even high—on certain minerals, it can cause low energy, hormone imbalances, an underperforming metabolism, and digestive issues. The best way to test mineral status and understand your individual needs is through a hair tissue mineral analysis (HTMA) test at your health practitioner's office, but adding in a daily mineral-rich drink or supplement is generally something I'd recommend for everyone wanting to improve their health. I've included recommendations for both in the resource section at the end of the workbook.

A healthy gut microbiome communicates with cells all over the body.

What You Need to Know

1. **Foods that damage the gut microbiome** include highly processed foods or foods that one would generally define as "junk food." No food is off limits here, but the reality is that many artificial ingredients in large quantities will damage the gut microbiome over time, especially if not balanced with whole foods. These include the following:
   - Canola, cottonseed, vegetable, sunflower, safflower, corn, and soybean oil.
   - Anything with high fructose corn syrup, soy protein, or soy flour.
   - Even "healthy" foods can be difficult for a damaged gut to digest, such as raw vegetables, chia seeds, nuts, and eggs.

2. **Other ways the gut can become damaged include** chronic infections from viruses, bacteria, fungi, or parasites; chronic stress; environmental toxins; low stomach acid; medications like hormonal birth control, NSAIDs (nonsteroidal anti-inflammatory drugs), PPIs (proton-pump inhibitors), and antibiotics; poor sleep; and nervous system dysregulation.

3. A great rule of thumb for a happy gut is simply to **eat a wide variety of plants** like vegetables, fruits, nuts, seeds, grains, beans, and legumes. A great goal is 21 different types of plants per week, but as a start, shoot for 5 per day!

4. **Making sure the body can absorb the foods and nutrients you're consuming to heal the gut is vital.** Drinking digestive bitters; chewing your food thoroughly; lightly cooking vegetables; soaking grains, seeds, and nuts; and giving the digestive system a 10- to 12-hour break every day are some simple ways to prep the body to absorb the nutrients it needs to restore gut health.

5. **Probiotics are healthy bacteria that populate your gut.** You can boost your probiotic consumption with fermented foods like sauerkraut, kimchi, raw pickles, kombucha, raw dairy products, homemade sourdough bread, miso, and tempeh—or you can take a spore-based probiotic. See the resources section on page 173 for my recommendations.

6. **Prebiotics are what probiotics eat to grow.** Prebiotics come in the form of fiber in foods like fruits, vegetables, starchy carbs, beans, legumes, nuts, and seeds. If grains, nuts, or seeds bother your stomach, try soaking or sprouting them first.

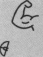

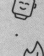

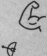

Activity: Reduce Gut Inflammation

Since your gut can't have a conversation with you, how do you know if you are experiencing gut health issues? Though this is something I suggest getting checked out by a health professional, and perhaps getting an HTMA or a gut-mapping test done, you can do some troubleshooting at home. Check off the symptoms that you experience regularly:

☐ diarrhea
☐ constipation
☐ gas/bloating
☐ irregular bowel movements
☐ reflux
☐ seasonal allergies
☐ anxiety/depression
☐ fatigue / brain fog
☐ trouble sleeping
☐ autoimmune disease

☐ acne, psoriasis, eczema, or rashes
☐ food intolerances/ sensitivities
☐ heart disease
☐ joint pain / muscle aches
☐ poor immune function
☐ seasonal allergies
☐ weight loss resistance / unexplained weight gain

If you marked one or more of these symptoms, it *could* be due to inflammation in the gut. Here are some easy steps to kick-start reducing gut inflammation and healing at home:

1. Remove or cut down on foods you know are causing damage.
2. Consume foods rich in probiotics and prebiotics daily to add new healthy bacteria.
3. Include bone broth, collagen, or gelatin daily to heal the lining of the gut.
4. Add in a daily mineral-rich drink. Many electrolyte drinks are on the market now that include the three macrominerals, sodium, potassium, and magnesium. All are essential for a healthy gut. I'll include my favorite electrolyte brands in the resource section.
5. If you frequently experience bloating, heartburn, or indigestion, add in a digestive bitters supplement before meals.

Activity: Daily Gut Check-In

Complete this check-in for a period of two weeks. For those who menstruate, because gut symptoms can also be tied to where you are in your menstrual cycle, it's better to begin tracking at least one week after your period has ended.

Date	Symptoms	Severity of symptoms	Where I'm at in my cycle (if it applies)	What I ate
	☐ bloating ☐ constipation ☐ diarrhea ☐ heartburn			
	☐ bloating ☐ constipation ☐ diarrhea ☐ heartburn			
	☐ bloating ☐ constipation ☐ diarrhea ☐ heartburn			
	☐ bloating ☐ constipation ☐ diarrhea ☐ heartburn			
	☐ bloating ☐ constipation ☐ diarrhea ☐ heartburn			
	☐ bloating ☐ constipation ☐ diarrhea ☐ heartburn			

Date	Symptoms	Severity of symptoms	Where I'm at in my cycle (if it applies)	What I ate
	☐ bloating ☐ constipation ☐ diarrhea ☐ heartburn			
	☐ bloating ☐ constipation ☐ diarrhea ☐ heartburn			
	☐ bloating ☐ constipation ☐ diarrhea ☐ heartburn			
	☐ bloating ☐ constipation ☐ diarrhea ☐ heartburn			
	☐ bloating ☐ constipation ☐ diarrhea ☐ heartburn			
	☐ bloating ☐ constipation ☐ diarrhea ☐ heartburn			
	☐ bloating ☐ constipation ☐ diarrhea ☐ heartburn			
	☐ bloating ☐ constipation ☐ diarrhea ☐ heartburn			

Reflection Questions

Are there foods you eat that you know consistently trigger digestive issues or breakouts? What kind of foods?

_____

_____

_____

_____

_____

_____

Reflecting on what you just learned, what are you doing currently to take care of your gut? What needs to change?

_____

_____

_____

_____

_____

_____

_____

Are there other patterns you've noticed, aside from eating certain foods, that trigger bloating, acid reflux, or digestive issues? Think about workouts, sleep, and stress.

_____

_____

_____

_____

_____

_____

PART TWO

Who Are You?

If you're frustrated with your current weight, energy levels, or how you look in a bikini, it's because you believe there's another version of you that's possible. You may doubt you can get there based on previous "failures." Despite those failures, there's something inside you that knows there's a different version of you who is confident, comfortable in your body, and probably lying poolside without a care in the world. And I call that version of you, YOU.

YOU is not the same as *you*. YOU is that supercharged version of yourself that deep down you know exists but just haven't been able to access quite yet. Discovering your YOU is ultimately what's going to drive your progress over the next year, and the vision work in this section will be your guiding light through the remainder of the workbook.

This is where we set the foundation in your mind before we start laying the bricks required to change your body. For each activity in this part, make sure you have at least half an hour of quiet, uninterrupted time. Begin by grounding or centering yourself with some deep breaths.

THE YOU MODEL

The YOU Model is a simple map of behavior. It looks at five elements: self-awareness, vision, beliefs, knowledge, and habits. It is based on the Neurological Levels model developed by Robert Dilts, a pioneer in the field of neurolinguistic programming.

We are taught that achieving a goal, like weight loss, looks something like this: set the goal; write it down; make sure it's specific, measurable, and achievable; and then create an action plan to move toward that goal. And while that is certainly not bad advice, it addresses only one aspect of behavior change—your habits. If you're someone who struggles with consistency, self-sabotage, or motivation, it's likely not that your willpower is weak but that you're not incorporating the other four elements of behavior change.

I would be willing to bet my car (which I really like) that you've never done the work you're about to do here in this section in a weight loss program before. And it's exactly why you're here. Commit to this work, and never go on a diet again.

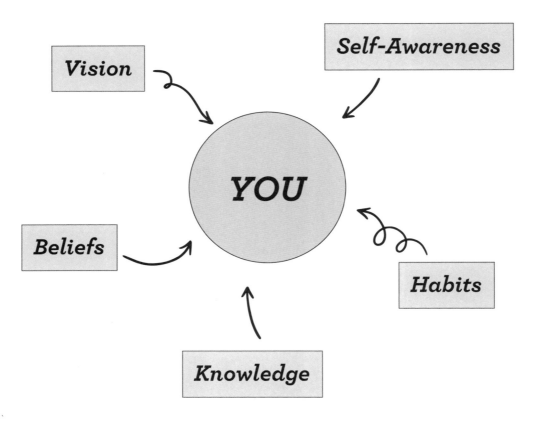

YOU *is not the same as* you*. YOU is that* supercharged version *of yourself that deep down* you know exists *but just haven't been able to* access *quite yet.*

Self-Awareness

Self-awareness is your ability to understand how your actions do or don't align with your goals.

Research suggests that those with strong self-awareness are more confident and make better decisions. Taking the time to pause and reflect—*without judgment*—on why you experience the shortcomings and challenges that you do means you can face new situations head-on with confidence. You won't become YOU on autopilot—it takes intention and the ability to see yourself clearly.

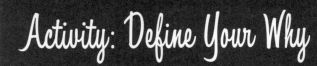

Activity: Define Your Why

Why do we do the things we do, buy the things we buy, or think the things we think? It's easy to just go about life doing, buying, thinking, and so on, but how often do you stop to think about the *why* behind it all? Finding your why will set you up with bite-sized motivation to use every single day to keep yourself going.

Where Are You Now?

Let's start by looking at where you're currently at. Answer the following questions with the first thing that pops into your head. We want to get that gut response.

What do my weekday and weekend meals look like?

_____

_____

What do I wear?

_____

_____

How do I move?

_____

_____

How do I sleep?

_____

_____

How do I feel?

_____

_____

How strong do I feel?

_____

_____

How do I play?

_____

_____

Where Do You Want to Be?

Next, let's look at your ideal: if every option was open to you, what would you choose? Again, answer from your gut. After, notice the discrepancies between the first round of questions and this one.

What do I want my weekday and weekend meals to look like?

_____

_____

What do I want to wear?

_____

_____

How do I want to move?

_____

_____

How do I want to sleep?

_____

_____

How do I want to feel?

_____

_____

How strong do I want to feel?

_____

_____

How do I want to play?

_____

_____

Why Do You Want That?

For each question, ask yourself *why* you want that. Then ask yourself why at least two more times, writing down whatever comes up. Dig deep here and get curious. Be as specific as possible! I know, this feels like a lot. But the point is to get at the core reason for your desire. Getting clear on why it is important to you will help you commit to making that a reality.

Example:

How do I want to sleep?
Answer: *For eight hours each night.*

Why do I want... that kind of sleep ?
Answer: *So I can feel rested.*

Why do I want... to feel rested ?
Answer: *When I feel rested, I make better decisions, I feel less stressed, and I don't yell at my kids.*

Now it's your turn. Ask why two more times for each question, starting with the following:

Why do I want my weekday and weekend meals to look like that?
Answer: _____

Why do I want... ?
Answer: _____

Why do I want... ?
Answer: _____

Why do I want to wear that?
Answer: _____

_____

Why do I want . . .   ?
Answer: _____

_____

Why do I want . . .   ?
Answer: _____

_____

_____

Why do I want to move like that?
Answer: _____

_____

Why do I want . . .   ?
Answer: _____

_____

Why do I want . . .   ?
Answer: _____

_____

_____

Why do I want that kind of sleep?
Answer: _____

_____

Why do I want . . .   ?
Answer: _____

_____

Why do I want . . .   ?
Answer: _____

_____

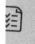
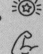
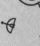

Why do I want to feel that way?
Answer: _____

_____

Why do I want . . . _____ ?
Answer: _____

Why do I want . . . _____ ?
Answer: _____

_____

Why do I want to feel that strong?
Answer: _____

Why do I want . . . _____ ?
Answer: _____

Why do I want . . . _____ ?
Answer: _____

_____

Why do I want to play that way?
Answer: _____

Why do I want . . . _____ ?
Answer: _____

Why do I want . . . _____ ?
Answer: _____

_____

Create Your Core Why

Notice any themes? Create one to three Core Why statements to help anchor them into your subconscious mind. These will serve as your North Star as you move on to the vision section, so spend some time here.

Example:

Perhaps you notice that several of your whys are anchored around wanting to be a better parent and more confident. Two Core Why statements might look like this:

Core Why

I prioritize my sleep and self-care so I can show up as my best self for my kids.

I prioritize doing things that make me feel confident, because when I feel confident, I genuinely feel more joy in my life.

Now create your own.

Core Why #1

Core Why #2

Core Why #3

Vision

Gone are the days where you wake up, catch a glimpse of your body in the mirror, and download WeightWatchers in a panic. You did this with good intentions, but that intention didn't have a true destination in mind. Sure, you might have said, "I want to lose 70 pounds." But what did that *look* like? What did it *feel* like? Who were *YOU as a person*? The 70-pounds-lighter version of you is not the same person you are today, so understanding that person is essential.

This is where your vision comes in. Vision is all about creating a crystal-clear idea of who you want to be. The more you can start to become that version of yourself today, the quicker you'll reach that destination.

If you are thinking, *I don't know what I'm eating for dinner tonight let alone who I want to be in a year,* you fit right in with the majority of women I work with. But this is why you spent time crafting your Core Why. When you understand your internal motivators, it begins to create new pathways in your brain that will slowly open up possibilities for the future that you may not have been able to see before. Do your best with this exercise, and know that you can return to it at any time throughout the year as your vision becomes clearer and clearer.

Vision is all about creating a crystal-clear idea of who you want to be.

Activity: Create Your Vision

You are more than just a number on a scale. Instead of a goal weight, let's envision what a healthy body feels and looks like to you. By using visualization (rather than just focusing on a number), you engage your senses, which makes the goal more embodied.

Begin by doing some freewriting on these questions:

If there were no limitations on what my body could do in a year, what would it look like? What would it feel like? What would it be able to do?

On a scale of 1–10, with 1 being the worst score (abysmal) and 10 being the best score (AH-MAZING), how do I rate each of the following areas?

① ② ③ ④ ⑤ ⑥ ⑦ ⑧ ⑨ ⑩   Love for my body

① ② ③ ④ ⑤ ⑥ ⑦ ⑧ ⑨ ⑩   Respect for my body

① ② ③ ④ ⑤ ⑥ ⑦ ⑧ ⑨ ⑩   How energized I feel in my body

① ② ③ ④ ⑤ ⑥ ⑦ ⑧ ⑨ ⑩   How I feel in my clothes

① ② ③ ④ ⑤ ⑥ ⑦ ⑧ ⑨ ⑩   How much fun I have in my body

① ② ③ ④ ⑤ ⑥ ⑦ ⑧ ⑨ ⑩   How strong I feel in my body

① ② ③ ④ ⑤ ⑥ ⑦ ⑧ ⑨ ⑩   Safety in my body

① ② ③ ④ ⑤ ⑥ ⑦ ⑧ ⑨ ⑩   Pain levels in my body

① ② ③ ④ ⑤ ⑥ ⑦ ⑧ ⑨ ⑩   My body's digestion

What would make each area a 10?

Love for my body: _____

_____

_____

_____

Respect for my body: _____

_____

_____

How energized I feel in my body:

How I feel in my clothes:

How much fun I have in my body:

How strong I feel in my body:

Safety in my body:

Pain levels in my body:

My body's digestion:

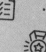

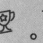

You should have a clear vision of the healthy YOU that you want to be. Inhabit this YOU, and start to look at every facet of their life. Answer the following questions as your YOU.

What does my morning and evening routine look like?

_____

_____

_____

_____

_____

_____

_____

_____

_____

_____

How well am I sleeping at night?

_____

_____

_____

_____

_____

_____

_____

_____

_____

How do I feel when I wake up in the morning?

_____

_____

_____

_____

_____

_____

_____

_____

How do I show up on a daily basis? What am I wearing? What are my priorities?

_____

_____

_____

_____

_____

_____

_____

_____

_____

What's my mood like?

_____

_____

_____

_____

_____

_____

How do I speak to myself?

_____

_____

_____

_____

_____

_____

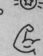

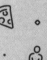

How worthy do I feel to be in my body?

_____
_____
_____
_____
_____
_____
_____
_____

How safe do I feel in my body?

_____
_____
_____
_____
_____
_____
_____
_____

How regulated is my nervous system? How often do I feel on edge, overwhelmed, reactive, or neurotic versus calm, cool, and collected?

_____
_____
_____
_____
_____
_____
_____
_____

How many times a week do I exercise? How often do I prioritize movement?

What is my digestion like?

What else comes up when I think about myself as this person? (Really paint a picture of who they are.)

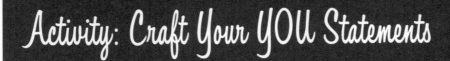

Activity: Craft Your YOU Statements

Using the vision you just created, craft some "YOU statements" to define the new YOU. You want these to be in present tense. Here are some examples to get you started:

- I am a person who gets back on track immediately. If I go out for nachos and margaritas, I simply return to my goals at the next meal instead of starting a bingefest.
- I am rarely hungover.
- I do my hair every day so I can be ready for anything.
- I am the type of person who easily makes it to the gym three days a week.
- I am a morning person.
- I don't do overwhelm.

I am ...

Here's the magic in this exercise. When you decide, for example, that you are a morning person, you are no longer just telling yourself to go to bed early or using your willpower to force it to happen. If you're a morning person, and that's just who YOU are, you will put more focus on doing things that will make you feel good in the morning.

Put your YOU statements into practice. You do not need to do every suggestion—choose what resonates. The point of this exercise is to begin to reprogram your subconscious. If you identify with being someone who is overweight, your subconscious mind will continually drive you to choose behaviors and thoughts that support this. If you identify as someone with a healthy, strong body, it will drive you to choose behaviors and thoughts to support this. But to reprogram yourself, it takes repeated exposure and embodiment of this new identity. Here are some ideas to get started:

☐ Write down your YOU statements on sticky notes and leave them around the house where you can see them.

☐ Set alarms throughout the day with different YOU statements.

☐ Record yourself repeating the statements on a voice recorder app and listen at least once per day.

☐ Choose one to three elements from your vision work to begin to incorporate into your life *now*. This can look like making a standing appointment for a blowout once a week, purchasing a larger water bottle to help you hydrate better, or downloading an app to lock your phone after 8:00 p.m. so you stop the scroll.

Beliefs

Neurolinguistic programming (NLP) is a way of changing thoughts and behaviors to help achieve desired outcomes. NLP considers beliefs to be mental representations of reality in that they shape thoughts, emotions, behaviors, and, most importantly, results. Because beliefs are based on past experiences (in other words, we have evidence to support our beliefs), they can either accelerate our progress on our goals or slow it down. Whatever beliefs you hold, you will subconsciously make decisions that support them.

The kinds of beliefs that slow us down are often called *limiting beliefs*. But even if you hold limiting beliefs that pump the brakes on your vision, YOU have the power to change them, meaning YOU also have the power to completely transform your life experience.

Here are some of the most common limiting beliefs I see while working with clients who are struggling with their weight.

- **"I self-sabotage."** This belief makes you think that no matter how well you're doing with sticking to a habit or moving toward your goal, you'll reverse all the progress you've made. You believe it's not a matter of *if* but *when* the other shoe will eventually drop.
- **"I always fail."** This belief states that you'll never achieve your goals no matter what, whether it's due to external or internal circumstances. You're just not good enough. This belief often holds people back from ever trying in the first place.
- **"I don't deserve it."** This belief often resides in the subconscious more than the conscious mind, but it's one that tells you that your goal is simply out of reach. It may be achievable for other people, but it's certainly not for you.
- **"If I stay where I'm at, I'll stay safe."** I see this manifest in two ways: (1) our primitive brain naturally holds the belief that if we are alive, we are safe, and therefore the safest option is to stay the same, even if a change is positive, or (2) many women hold a deep-seated belief that looking a certain way will protect them from unwanted advances from men, especially if they are survivors of sexual assault.

If you believe you're a self-sabotager, you'll subconsciously make decisions that support this belief. If you believe you're a failure at weight loss, you'll subconsciously make decisions that support that belief. But on the other hand, if you believe you're a person who doesn't break promises to themselves, and your body is becoming more metabolically healthy every day, then you better bet you'll subconsciously make decisions that support this belief too!

Whatever beliefs you hold, you will subconsciously make decisions that support them.

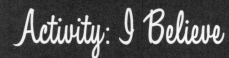

Activity: I Believe

Return to your vision and highlight any of the YOU statements that feel uncomfy, impossible, or hard instead of fun and exciting. *Why* do you feel this way? These whys are your Core Limiting Beliefs.

Example:

YOU statement that feels out of reach: *I am a morning person.*

Why does it feel out of reach? *I can't remember a time in my life when I didn't hit snooze. I have no evidence that I can be a morning person, and it feels out of reach.*

Your turn:

YOU statement that feels out of reach:

Why does it feel out of reach?

YOU statement that feels out of reach:

Why does it feel out of reach?

YOU statement that feels out of reach: _____

_____

Why does it feel out of reach? _____

_____

_____

_____

_____

YOU statement that feels out of reach: _____

_____

Why does it feel out of reach? _____

_____

_____

_____

_____

YOU statement that feels out of reach: _____

_____

Why does it feel out of reach? _____

_____

_____

_____

_____

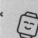

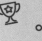

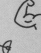

Next, make a list of reasons you hold these beliefs. All the reasons you write down are also Core Limiting Beliefs that you hold—sneaky, right? Some examples might include the following:

- I don't deserve _____ because _____ .
- This isn't going to work for me because _____ .
- This hasn't worked in the past for me, so it won't work now because _____ .

Core Limiting Beliefs

Note: You could spend an hour on each Core Limiting Belief, so it's okay if you don't get this all done at once. This is deep work, and I'm so proud of you for sticking with it. You are changing your brain, and this will impact not only your life but the lives of your loved ones, especially your children, if you have them.

Imagine your Core Limiting Beliefs as a chair. The seat of the chair is your belief, and the legs of the chair are your reasons for holding that belief. When you dismantle the reasons or evidence of a Core Limiting Belief, the belief loses its power.

Take the legs off the chair by asking yourself these questions:

How did I come to believe these beliefs? Have I always believed them?

_____

_____

_____

If I were under oath and were asked if these beliefs were factual, what would I say?

_____

_____

_____

Has there ever been an instance where these beliefs didn't apply in my life?

_____

_____

_____

Where will I be in one, five, or ten years by continuing to hold these beliefs?

_____

_____

_____

If my child or best friend held these same beliefs, what would I tell them?

_____

_____

_____

What are one or two small steps I can take today to begin to wear these new beliefs I have about myself?

_____

_____

_____

Knowledge

It's great to tell yourself you need to eat more protein and get to the gym, but *do you know why*? Truly knowing why eating 30 grams of protein for breakfast and lifting weights helps you achieve your goals is a subconscious understanding. We don't like being told "eat the protein because I said so"; though it may work on your four-year-old from time to time, it doesn't work on you after the initial excitement of a new program wears off. Understanding your body and metabolism makes decision-making easier.

The good news? We already explored the knowledge piece of the puzzle in part 1! Of course, there is much more to understand about how the body works, so if you're interested to learn more, I've included some of my favorite educational books, podcasts, and websites here. For even more resources, check the resource section at the end of the workbook.

Understanding your body and metabolism makes decision-making easier.

Activity: More Research

Return to your YOU statements in the vision section, and make a list of topics you'd like to learn more about and where you'll start. I'll make a list of some of my favorite resources surrounding each pillar of the Metabolic Ecosystem to help. And if you'd like something that captures all of the following, check out my book *Metabolism Makeover*.

Blood Sugar Control

- ☐ *Good Energy: The Surprising Connection Between Metabolism and Limitless Health* by Dr. Casey Means

Muscle

- ☐ *Forever Strong: A New, Science-Based Strategy for Aging Well* by Dr. Gabrielle Lyon
- ☐ *Muscle Science for Women* podcast

Movement

- ☐ Nutritious Movement (www.nutritiousmovement.com)
- ☐ *Move Your DNA: Restore Your Health Through Natural Movement* by Katy Bowman

Sleep

- ☐ *Why We Sleep: Unlocking the Power of Sleep and Dreams* by Matthew Walker
- ☐ *The Sleep Revolution: Transforming Your Life, One Night at a Time* by Arianna Huffington

Stress Management

- ☐ *The Calm Mom Podcast*
- ☐ *The 5 Resets: Rewire Your Brain and Body for Less Stress and More Resilience* by Dr. Aditi Nerurkar

> **Gut Health**
>
> ☐ *Fiber Fueled: The Plant-Based Gut Health Program for Losing Weight, Restoring Your Health, and Optimizing Your Microbiome* by Will Bulsiewicz
>
> ☐ *The Good Gut: Taking Control of Your Weight, Your Mood, and Your Long-Term Health* by Justin Sonnenburg and Erica Sonnenburg

Say, for example, you're only sleeping six hours per night, but YOU consistently get in a solid eight. What books, podcasts, or trainings can you look at to help support this goal? If you have consistent digestion issues, but YOU are rarely bloated and have regular bowel movements, is it time to look into working with a functional practitioner who can do a gut map and see what might be going on under the hood?

Habits

Several studies show that about 45 percent of your day is driven by habits. So you can imagine your daily habits are a pretty significant part of YOU. But habits are difficult to change because humans are always striving for equilibrium. Ever notice that even when you have the best intention for habit change, *something* always ends up sabotaging those intentions? It's because an alarm goes off in our brain when we try to make a change! And the bigger the change, the more our bodies fight back. This is why I like to place an emphasis on micro habits over macro habits—which you'll see when you get to part 3. The smaller the change, the more likely you are to seamlessly integrate that change into your daily routine.

A habit you can start strengthening right now is your consistency. Losing motivation is 100 percent normal, especially when the thing we're doing isn't always fun. While motivation is a desire, consistency is an act. You have to learn how to bring discipline on board when motivation is wavering, because discipline drives consistency, and discipline is a learned behavior. And just like any other habit, it requires daily practice and repetition.

When you experience this:	*Do this:*
Feeling like a habit is too overwhelming or is making your life more difficult than easy.	• Ask yourself if you can break that habit down into a smaller habit, a.k.a. a micro habit (we'll learn all about these in part 3). • Remove barriers that are making your habit difficult.
Having a hard time remembering your habit.	• Create a daily standing meeting with yourself, even if it is *not* a daily habit. • Set up automations.
Wanting to give up.	Revisit your Core Why.
Struggling with consistency and can't figure out why.	Revisit your YOU statements to remind your subconscious who the heck you are.
Finding you don't have time for your habit.	Set aside time every weekend to get organized for the week. The Weekly Review/Preview in part 4 will help with this.
Experiencing any or all of the above.	Find an accountability partner.

Here are some examples if you need more help.

Break a larger habit down to a smaller habit. If you are currently struggling with a macro habit, like going to the gym five days a week, try breaking it down into a micro habit. A micro habit could look like this:

- Going to the gym two days per week.
- Bringing gym clothes with you to work and changing into them at 4:00 p.m.
- Committing to any form of movement five days per week instead of going to the gym.

Remove barriers.

- Remove foods from your pantry that require a lot of willpower to not overconsume.
- Meditate in your car if there are too many distractions at home.
- Get rid of the idea that you can't walk or work out at home in your regular clothes if you hate changing into workout clothes.

Create a daily standing meeting with yourself, even if the focus changes from day to day. If you go to the gym at 5:00 p.m. on Monday and Thursday, on the other days during that time, commit to a different kind of movement. For example, come home and walk, stretch, or squeeze in a quick yoga session.

Set up automations.

- Set an alarm on your phone to remind you to do that habit at a particular time.
- Put meal delivery on autoship.
- Set your blue-light blockers on the kitchen counter every morning and set a reminder to put them on at 7:00 p.m.
- Download an app that locks your phone at a certain time so you stop the scroll.

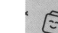

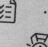

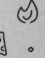

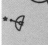

Revisit your YOU statements to remind your subconscious who the heck YOU are. You may even decide to add a few more statements based on whatever habits you're struggling with, such as any of these statements:

- I treat my body like the temple that it is.
- I am the strongest I've ever been.
- I take care of my body, and it takes care of me.

Get organized every week.

- Schedule time to meal prep.
- Add workouts and walks to your calendar.
- Set up automations, like weekly meal delivery.

Find an accountability partner. Here's what I know from working with over eight thousand clients: you are 96 percent more likely to achieve a goal if you both have someone holding you accountable and have a set time and place to check in regularly. I bet you can think of someone in your life who wants to go on a similar journey or would love to support you in this way. But if not, another way to go about this is to join Metabolism Makeover, our online community where you are held accountable and can receive coaching and personalized feedback by our team of dietitians. You will also have access to videos of me walking you through the entire Metabolism Makeover method step by step. You can join on my website at metabolismmakeover.co or by scanning the QR code below.

Activity: Build Up Your Habits

Think about something you've been wanting to make a habit, but you've been struggling to make it happen. Using the chart below, pinpoint why it's been a struggle and come up with one or two actions you can take toward becoming more consistent today.

HABIT YOU'RE STRUGGLING WITH	WHY IT'S BEEN A STRUGGLE	ACTION STEPS

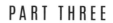

PART THREE

Your Four-Week Jump Start

Now that you have knowledge of how your body's metabolism works and what's required to lose weight for good, you're ready to take action!
"But when should I start?"

I encourage you to begin *now*! There is no need to wait until the first of the month or three months from now when "things slow down" (they won't). It's important to begin to shift your thinking from "I'm starting a new diet program next month to lose X pounds" to "I'm supporting my body and my metabolism daily because I love myself."

I do recommend starting on a Monday and taking a couple of days to plan prior to jumping in.

THE FIRST FOUR WEEKS

For the first four weeks, you'll be doing two things:

1. Implementing a new micro habit each week
2. Evaluating your week using the Weekly Review/Preview process to help support self-awareness

Micro habits: Each of the first four weeks, I'll introduce a new micro habit. These are my four most potent, effective habits that my clients consistently see real success with while making over their metabolism and getting quick wins. You will focus on one micro habit in week 1, then stack the second micro habit in week 2, the third in week 3, and then by week 4, you will be implementing four new micro habits. The following pages will help you track these habits.

			Eat the right amount of carbs
		Take a 20-minute power walk	Take a 20-minute power walk
	Eat PHFF at every meal	Eat PHFF at every meal	Eat PHFF at every meal
Eat 30 g of protein at breakfast	Eat 30 g of protein at breakfast	Eat 30 g of protein at breakfast	Eat 30 g of protein at breakfast
WEEK 1	WEEK 2	WEEK 3	WEEK 4

Weekly Review/Preview: Each week, you'll complete a Weekly Review/Preview process designed to increase your self-awareness around your day-to-day actions. Because here's the deal: modern life is stressful. It's easy to go on autopilot and not notice how you feel, how you're getting in your own way, or how your choices are supporting (or sabotaging) your vision. This process will give you a clearer picture of various factors that impact your metabolism as well as what's working and what's not working so you can make adjustments.

Each week, you'll choose a day to complete your Review/Preview. I recommend doing this on Saturday or Sunday before you typically do any kind of setup for your week, like grocery shopping, meal prepping, or checking your calendar to see what's going on that week. Before week 1, you'll complete the Metabolic Movers activity on page 71 instead of a Review. For all the other weeks, you will use the Review as you preview your next week to help inform changes you may need to make.

For example, during your Review, you might realize you got only six hours of sleep three nights this week. Think about what steps you need to take to get seven or more hours the next week, based on what your schedule looks like.

Get Your Baseline with Metabolic Movers

Before we move into the Four-Week Jump Start, it's important to establish a starting point with your metabolism. The following chart offers insight into where your metabolism is currently at, and in week 4 you'll be able to see how the micro habits you've implemented are moving the metabolic needle.

Right now, before you start, take an assessment of these. Feel free to add a few of your own measurements in the blank spaces at the end of the chart. At the end of week 4, I'll direct you to come back here and update the chart so you can see the magic at work!

Here's a code you can use:

1 = 5–7 times/week	2 = 3–5 times/week	3 = 1–2 times/week	4 = rarely/never

	BEFORE WEEK 1	AFTER WEEK 4
How often do I have cravings?		
How often do I feel hangry?		
How often am I eating to the point of discomfort?		
How often do I *not* have a bowel movement?		
How often do I experience bloating?		
How often do I eat less than 30 g protein at a meal?		
How often do I feel tired and sluggish most of the day?		
How many days per week do I feel highly stressed?		
How often do I get less than 7 hours of sleep?		
How confident do I feel? ☺ = confident, 😐 = semi-confident, ☹ = not confident	☺ 😐 ☹	☺ 😐 ☹

Ditch the Scale, and Use Photos Instead

Taking photos is essential—do not skip this step. If you don't see the immediate results on the scale, you'll want to make sure you're tracking the changes to your body! Oftentimes when eating for your metabolism, you'll start to gain muscle and lose fat, and that won't necessarily be reflected on the scale. Take front- and side-facing photos in front of your mirror to track progress, and make sure your clothing and lighting remain consistent. If you menstruate, know that where you're at in your menstrual cycle will impact the photos, so it's a good idea to take them around the same time in your cycle. Keep photos in a folder on your phone.

Begin now! *There is no need to wait until "things slow down" (they won't).*

Reflection Questions

Before week 1:

What is your biggest fear going into this, and why?

_____

_____

Write your Core Why and YOU statements here to remind yourself who the heck YOU are!

_____

_____

_____

_____

After week 4:

Which habit was the easiest for you to implement?

_____

_____

Which habit was most challenging for you? How can you make changes in the future to make it easier for yourself?

_____

_____

_____

_____

_____

What are you most proud of this month?

_____

_____

_____

WHAT YOU NEED TO KNOW BEFORE GETTING STARTED

The following are some incredibly important questions that always pop up before getting started in your metabolism makeover! You will want to bookmark this page as several of these questions are bound to pop up over the next four weeks.

How do I know how much to eat if I'm not tracking calories?

Believe it or not, we did not evolve to have to use an app to track our food and maintain our weight. Our bodies have built-in calorie counters in the form of our hunger and satiety hormones! I suggest putting away the calorie or macro tracker for the first four weeks. Instead, become aware of the protein, healthy fat, fiber, and starchy carb amounts you're eating at each meal, and make sure you can go about four hours between meals without becoming ravenous. You can always go back to tracking, but part of this method is learning how to reconnect with your body and interpret the signals it is sending you.

What if eating protein, healthy fat, and fiber at every meal isn't keeping me full for four hours?

A simple way to gauge whether you are eating enough at meals is the ability to go about four hours before needing food again. If your meals are not keeping you satisfied for four hours, here is what to do next:

1. Add 10 more grams of protein.
2. Increase fiber to at least 8 grams for that meal.
3. Add 10 grams of fat.

Start with protein, then move to fiber, then fat. Take a look at the following two examples:

If your 8:00 a.m. smoothie has 30 grams of protein, 1 tablespoon of almond butter, 1 tablespoon of chia seeds, and ½ cup of raspberries, but you stay full only until 10:00 a.m., it's time to add more food. Start with adding more protein, and if that doesn't do the trick, evaluate the fiber (in this case, the smoothie already has more than 8 grams of fiber), and then add another serving of fat.

If your 12:00 p.m. salad at lunch has grilled chicken, spring mix, cherry tomatoes, a hard-boiled egg, 1 ounce of cheddar cheese, and 2 tablespoons of dressing, but you're getting hungry at 2:30, it's time to add more food. Start by adding another ounce of chicken or another hard-boiled egg, and if that doesn't keep you full until at least 4:00 p.m., look at how much fiber is in your salad. Believe it or not, salads are often lacking in fiber! This one would have only 1–2 grams. You can bulk up the fiber by adding broccoli, cauliflower, or artichoke, and if that doesn't do the trick, add an extra serving of fat that also contains fiber, such as ½ avocado, 10 olives, or 2 tablespoons sunflower seeds.

What if I need a snack to hold me over?

It's incredibly normal to need a snack, especially when you're going more than four hours between meals! Common snacks are high in low-fiber starchy carbohydrates, like chips and popcorn. Even fruit, which I encourage you to eat, when eaten by itself, will cause blood sugar to rise and crash quickly, leaving you hungry within an hour.

Snacks will be variable based on your hunger and how long they will need to sustain you until your next meal. You'll find a snack chart on page 87.

Can I still go out to eat?

Of course you can still go out to eat! My favorite dining-out hack? *Choose one starchy carb.* If you really want a burger and fries, decide if you'd prefer the fries or the bun on the burger. Do a bunless burger and fries or a regular burger with a veggie side. Out for Italian food? Choose bread *or* pasta. This way, you can enjoy your favorite foods without all-or-nothing thinking.

Friday pizza night isn't exactly blood sugar friendly or high protein, but it's a family tradition. What do I do?

There's always a way to make meals blood sugar friendly. Just think PHFF. Maybe you do a thin crust pizza (fewer carbs!), add extra protein on top, and make a big side salad (fiber!). Maybe every other week you make pizzas at home so you have more control. Or perhaps you do a big salad with

grilled chicken and make a slice of pizza the side dish instead of the main attraction.

For more "What do I do when _____?" questions like these, there is a framework on page 118 that can help you with your decision-making.

Can I still drink alcohol?

Yes, you can still drink alcohol. Here is what you need to know about alcohol and your metabolism: the body always prioritizes clearing alcohol, which is technically a toxin, from your system over your metabolism. So help your body out by skipping sweetened mixers, sugary wines, liqueurs, and high-carb beers. No-sugar mixers with hard liquor and clean, low-sugar wines are best. Ask for club soda instead of tonic or regular soda. Or try a margarita with tequila, orange liqueur, fresh lime, and no agave.

What foods can't I eat?

Great news—no foods are off limits! This method isn't about cutting out certain foods, as long as you're controlling your blood sugar and eating foods that make you feel good.

What if I'm vegetarian or vegan?

I still want you to eat 30 grams of protein for breakfast, but if you find it challenging to hit 30 grams at every meal, that's okay! Blood sugar balance is still important. Be mindful of your starchy carbs, include some form of protein at each meal, and really focus on fiber and healthy fats to control blood sugar and stay full.

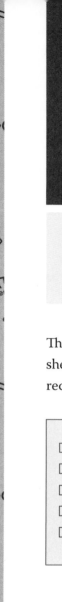

Week One

MICRO HABIT: *Eat 30 grams of protein at breakfast*

Why it matters: Protein is your key macronutrient when it comes to keeping you full, revving up your metabolism, and getting you lean. A high-protein breakfast has been shown to reduce overall calories throughout the day.

There are so many ways to get protein in, but to get you started, here is a little cheat sheet of common breakfast proteins and a few simple, quick, and delicious breakfast recipes and ideas. On page 79, you can record your breakfasts each day.

- ☐ eggs (6 grams per egg)
- ☐ cottage cheese (28 grams per cup)
- ☐ protein powder (see label)
- ☐ Greek yogurt (23 grams per cup)
- ☐ turkey bacon (5 grams per slice)
- ☐ chicken sausage (16 grams per 4 ounces)
- ☐ ground turkey (30 grams per 4 ounces)
- ☐ milk (8 grams per cup)

RECIPES

Blackberry chia pudding (makes 2)

2 cups unsweetened nut milk

1 cup blackberries

½ tsp vanilla extract

2 servings (~25 grams of protein per serving) vanilla protein powder

¼ cup chia seeds

¼ cup sliced almonds

1. Add all the ingredients except the almonds to a bowl and mix until well incorporated.
2. Divide into two smaller containers, cover, and refrigerate overnight.
3. Top with almonds before eating in the morning.

Peanut butter banana smoothie (makes 1)

1 cup unsweetened nut milk
1 serving (~25 grams of protein per serving) vanilla protein powder
1½ tbsp all-natural peanut butter
½ small banana, frozen
1 tbsp chia seeds

Add all ingredients to a blender and blend until smooth.

Feta egg scramble (makes 1)

3 eggs
2 tbsp crumbled feta cheese
⅓ cup cottage cheese
1 tsp fresh dill
sea salt and black pepper, to taste
1 tsp olive oil
¾ cup halved cherry tomatoes
¾ cup berries of your choice

1. In a small bowl, whisk the eggs. Stir in the feta, cottage cheese, dill, salt, and pepper until well combined.
2. Heat the oil in a skillet over medium heat. Add the halved tomatoes and cook for about two minutes, until softened. Pour the egg mixture into the pan and cook, stirring to scramble the eggs, to your desired doneness.
3. Serve with a side of berries.

PB&J yogurt bowl (makes 1)

1 cup 2% plain Greek yogurt
1 tbsp honey
2 tbsp all-natural peanut butter
½ cup strawberries

Add the yogurt and honey to a serving bowl and mix to combine. Top with the peanut butter and strawberries.

Pizza omelet (makes 1)

3 eggs
sea salt and black pepper, to taste
1 tsp butter
1 cup baby spinach
2 tbsp marinara sauce
1 oz mozzarella
7 pepperoni slices
2 tbsp sliced black olives
2 tbsp finely chopped fresh basil, optional

1. In a small bowl, whisk together the eggs, sea salt, and black pepper until frothy.
2. Melt the butter in a skillet over medium heat. Add the spinach and cook until just wilted, then pour the egg mixture into the skillet and let it cook until almost set. Place the spinach, marinara, mozzarella, pepperoni, and olives on one half of the omelet and then fold the other half over on top. Transfer the omelet onto a plate.
3. Top with basil, if using, and serve.

Preview Week One

What's happening this week:

_____

_____

_____

_____

_____

_____

Do a little brain dump of everything you've got going on this week. Dinners out, lunch meetings, soccer practice, date nights, meetings. Look at your calendar and lay it all out.

How to navigate obstacles:

_____

_____

_____

_____

_____

_____

How will early, rushed mornings impact breakfast? What about Sunday brunch? What's your plan? If you prepare breakfast the night before, are there things on your schedule that could make that difficult?

Here are some examples:

*Early morning meeting: Prep breakfast the night before. Make sure it's something you can eat in the car.

*Sunday brunch: Look at the menu ahead of time, and seek out high-protein options.

*A couple of late nights: Prep breakfasts for the week on Sunday so you don't have to think about it all week.

Checklist:

☐ Plan out your breakfasts for the week using the recipes in this section or by thinking about your normal breakfast and adding enough protein to hit 30 grams.

☐ Write out your planned meals using the chart in this section.

☐ Check to make sure you have enough protein on hand. If not, add it to your grocery list.

☐ Meal prep breakfasts ahead of time, if necessary. Most recipes are for one to two servings but could be doubled or tripled.

☐ Track your progress.

TRACK YOUR PROGRESS

I suggest planning your breakfasts out for the week here, but if you prefer, you can add them after you've already eaten them.

DATE/DAY OF THE WEEK	30 GRAMS OF PROTEIN FOR BREAKFAST

Review Week One

How many days did I stick
to my micro habit?

1 2 3 4 5 6 7

How many days did I sleep
seven or more hours?

1 2 3 4 5 6 7

How many days was I able to last at
least four hours between meals?

1 2 3 4 5 6 7

How were my confidence
levels this week?

Low   Average   High

How were my energy levels?

Low   Average   High

How were my stress levels?

Low   Average   High

Did I experience any digestive issues
or bloating this week? ☐ Yes ☐ No

Notes:

Did I experience cravings or
hangriness this week? ☐ Yes ☐ No

Notes:

What went well this week? What am I proud of?

What was a struggle?

Changes I'll make for next week:

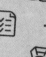
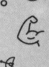

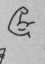

Week Two

MICRO HABIT: *Eat protein, healthy fat, and fiber (PHFF) at every meal*

Why it matters: Last week, we established the importance of protein at breakfast, so now it's time to introduce the other two potent blood sugar modulators: healthy fat and fiber. As a recap, both fat and fiber lessen the blood sugar response when eating foods that contain carbohydrates. When we have steady blood sugar, the body is able to switch from burning carbohydrates to burning fat for energy more easily. When we have blood sugar spikes and crashes (from eating carbs alone), the large insulin response that occurs blocks fat burning and causes cravings, increased hunger, and energy dips.

Here are some sample groceries and easy recipes that focus on PHFF to get you started.

SAMPLE GROCERY LIST

Proteins:
- [ ] rotisserie chicken
- [ ] ground beef
- [ ] canned tuna
- [ ] salmon
- [ ] eggs
- [ ] 2% Greek yogurt

Healthy fats:
- [ ] shredded cheese
- [ ] avocado
- [ ] nut butter
- [ ] olive oil
- [ ] black olives

Fiber and starchy carbs:
- [ ] carrots, broccoli, lettuce, tomatoes, cucumbers
- [ ] raspberries, apples
- [ ] chia seeds
- [ ] black beans
- [ ] sweet potato fries
- [ ] quinoa
- [ ] red lentil pasta
- [ ] high-fiber crackers (at least 3 grams per serving)

Extras:
- [ ] marinara
- [ ] preferred seasonings

SAMPLE MEALS

The following meals are not recipes and do not contain serving sizes. This is done to show how simple it is to combine PHFF in meals throughout the week without recipes. Serving sizes look different for everyone, so use the charts on pages 84–87 to see how much PHFF to start with in a meal. If meals are not keeping you full at least four hours, refer to the guide on page 74 to know what to add to your meal.

Note: I have used the same breakfast during the week for reducing decision fatigue and for meal prep purposes, but you can have a different type of breakfast every day if you prefer!

	MON	TUES	WED	THURS	FRI	SAT	SUN
Breakfast	Greek yogurt, nut butter, chia seeds, and raspberries					Scrambled eggs with avocado + apple slices	
Lunch	Egg salad made with mashed avocado + carrots + high-fiber crackers		Taco bowls with black beans, tomato, lettuce, cheddar cheese, rotisserie chicken, and avocado		Salmon + quinoa + cucumber, tomato, olive, and olive oil salad	Red lentil pasta with tuna, olive oil, black olives, cucumbers, and tomatoes	Lunch out!
Dinner	Red lentil pasta + meat sauce and broccoli	Taco bowls with black beans, tomato, lettuce, cheddar cheese, rotisserie chicken, and avocado	Bunless cheeseburger with lettuce and tomatoes + sweet potato fries	Salmon + quinoa + cucumber, tomato, olive, and olive oil salad	Red lentil pasta with tuna, olive oil, black olives, cucumbers, and tomatoes	Dinner out!	Leftover protein + leftover veggies + avocado or cheese

The following charts give you an easy breakdown of where to start for breakfast, lunch, and dinner, as well as smoothies and snacks. The top of each column tells you how much of each item (protein, healthy fat, fiber, and starchy carbs) to choose, and you can mix and match as much as you like. And if you enjoyed your breakfasts from week 1, it's more than okay to continue eating those. In week 4, you will learn the exact amount of starchy carbs to eat for your body, but for now, go ahead and add them in as you typically eat them. For example, if you always have a starch at dinner, choose one for dinner. If you don't normally have a starch at lunch, go ahead and leave it out. Also, note that for the starchy carbs, the amounts offered are estimates. Be sure to check the packaging for exact amounts.

Find a blank chart on page 89 for you to record your meals each day.

BREAKFAST			
PROTEIN (1)	HEALTHY FAT (1–3)	FIBER (2–3)	STARCHY CARBS, OPTIONAL (30–40 G CARBS)
◆ 3 eggs + 1 scoop collagen powder ◆ 3 eggs + 3 pieces bacon ◆ 2 eggs + 2 oz chicken sausage ◆ 2 eggs + 2 egg whites + 1 scoop collagen ◆ 2 eggs + 2 oz steak ◆ 1 cup plain Greek yogurt + 10 g collagen ◆ 1 cup cottage cheese + 10 g collagen	◆ ½ cup sliced avocado ◆ 2 tsp avocado, olive, or coconut oil ◆ 1 tbsp butter ◆ 3 tbsp pumpkin seeds ◆ 3 tbsp nuts (walnuts, almonds, pistachios, peanuts, pecans, etc.)	◆ 1 cup nonstarchy vegetables (see "lunch and dinner" for examples) ◆ 1 cup most fruits ◆ ½ cup blackberries or raspberries ◆ 1 tbsp chia seeds ◆ 1 tbsp acacia fiber	◆ 2 pieces whole-grain, sprouted, or sourdough bread ◆ ⅓ cup uncooked steel-cut oats ◆ 2 tortillas ◆ ¾ cup diced potatoes ◆ 1 English muffin ◆ 1 serving pancakes (whole-grain, grain-free, or high-protein pancake mixes) ◆ 2–3 waffles (whole-grain, grain-free, or high-protein waffles)

Both **fat** *and* **fiber** *lessen the* **blood sugar response** *when eating foods that contain* **carbohydrates***.*

LUNCH			
PROTEIN (1)	**HEALTHY FAT (1–3)**	**FIBER (UNLIMITED)**	**STARCHY CARBS, OPTIONAL (30–40 G)**

• 3.5 oz cooked chicken breast
• 4 oz ground chicken or turkey
• 6 oz nitrate-free deli turkey
• 4 oz cooked 90% lean ground beef
• 4.5 oz cooked salmon
• 5 oz canned tuna
• 6 oz shrimp or 4.5 oz cooked shrimp
• 1 cup cottage cheese
	• 1 oz cheese
	• ½ avocado, sliced
	• 1 tbsp mayo
	• 2 tsp olive or avocado oil
	• 1 tbsp butter
	• ½ cup hummus
	• 1 tbsp pesto
	• ⅓ cup guacamole
		• nonstarchy vegetables such as:
		  ◇ asparagus
		  ◇ broccoli
		  ◇ bell peppers
		  ◇ cabbage
		  ◇ carrots
		  ◇ cauliflower
		  ◇ cucumbers
		  ◇ green beans
		  ◇ spinach
			• ¼ cup uncooked or ⅔ cup cooked rice (white, brown, wild)
			• 2 servings crackers
			• 2 pieces whole-grain, sprouted, or sourdough bread
			• 2 oz lentil or chickpea pasta
			• ¾ cup baby red potatoes
			• ⅔ cup quinoa
			• ¼ cup uncooked or ¾ cup cooked lentils
			• ¾ cup chickpeas
			• 2 small tortillas

DINNER			
PROTEIN (1)	**HEALTHY FAT (1–3)**	**FIBER (UNLIMITED)**	**STARCHY CARBS, OPTIONAL (30–40 G)**

• 3.5 oz cooked chicken breast
• 4 oz cooked chicken thighs
• 4 oz ground chicken or turkey
• 4 oz cooked 90% lean ground beef
• 4 oz cooked sirloin
• 4.5 oz cooked salmon
• 4 oz cooked cod, halibut, or tilapia
• 4.5 oz cooked shrimp
• 5 oz cooked scallops
• 4 oz cooked pork chops or tenderloin
	• 1 oz cheese
	• ¼ cup sour cream
	• 1 tbsp butter
	• ½ avocado, sliced
	• ⅓ cup guacamole
	• 2 tsp olive or avocado oil
	• 20 large olives
	• 1 tbsp pesto
		• nonstarchy vegetables such as:
		  ◇ artichoke
		  ◇ asparagus
		  ◇ broccoli
		  ◇ brussels sprouts
		  ◇ bell peppers
		  ◇ carrots
		  ◇ cauliflower
		  ◇ eggplant
		  ◇ green beans
		  ◇ greens (spinach, collards, kale, romaine)
		  ◇ mushrooms
		  ◇ okra
		  ◇ onion
		  ◇ radishes
		  ◇ squash
		  ◇ tomatoes
		  ◇ zucchini
			• 1 cup cooked corn
			• 1¼ cups cooked peas
			• ¼ cup uncooked or ⅔ cup cooked rice (white, brown, wild)
			• 2 small tortillas
			• ¼ cup uncooked or ¾ cup cooked lentils
			• 2 pieces whole-grain, sprouted, or sourdough bread
			• 2 oz dry lentil or chickpea pasta
			• ¾ cup baby red potatoes
			• ¼ cup uncooked or ⅔ cup cooked quinoa

When we have **steady blood sugar,** *the body is able to switch from burning carbohydrates to burning fat for energy* **more easily**.

SMOOTHIE		
PROTEIN (1)	**HEALTHY FAT (1–3)**	**FIBER (2–3)**
• 30 g protein powder • 30 g collagen powder • 20 g protein powder + 10 g collagen powder • 1 cup plain Greek yogurt • 1 cup cottage cheese	• 3 tbsp canned coconut milk (unsweetened) • 2 tbsp coconut flakes (unsweetened) • 2 tbsp heavy cream • ½ cup avocado, sliced • 2 tsp coconut oil • 2 tbsp hemp seeds • 1 tbsp nut butter (almond, cashew, peanut)	• 1 tbsp chia seeds • 1 tbsp acacia fiber • 2 tsp inulin fiber • 1 tbsp flax seeds • 1 cup frozen cauliflower rice • 1 cup shredded carrot • 2 cups spinach • 2 tbsp cacao powder • ½ cup blackberries or raspberries

SNACKS		
PROTEIN (1–2, 15–20 G)	**FAT (1)**	**OPTIONAL ADD-ONS**
• ¾ cup cottage cheese • 1 cup plain Greek yogurt • 25–20 g protein powder • 2 beef sticks • 3 hard-boiled eggs • 2 string cheese sticks	• ⅓ cup guacamole • 3 tbsp pumpkin seeds • ½ cup sliced avocado • 1 tbsp nut butter (almond, cashew, peanut) • 2 tbsp nuts • 20 olives	• nonstarchy vegetables • 1 serving crackers • ½ cup berries • 2–3 rice cakes • 1 serving tortilla chips • 1 tbsp chia seeds

*Remember, **serving sizes** look different for everyone.*

Preview Week Two

What's happening this week:

_____
_____
_____
_____
_____
_____

Do a little brain dump of everything you've got going on this week. Dinners out, lunch meetings, soccer practice, date nights, meetings. Look at your calendar and lay it all out.

How to navigate obstacles:

_____
_____
_____
_____
_____
_____

How will three soccer practices this week impact dinner? How about the lunch meetings—do you have control over what you'll eat or not? If so, what's your plan? If not, what's your plan?

Here are some examples:
*For three soccer practices: Prep a couple of proteins, vegetables, and starchy carbs to make it easy to combine for dinners.
*Lunch meetings: Look at the menu ahead of time and seek out high-protein options that include vegetables for fiber.

_____
_____
_____

Checklist:

☐ Plan out breakfasts, lunches, and dinners for the week using the charts on pages 84–87 by thinking about your normal lunch and dinner and seeing how you can edit those to fit PHFF.

☐ Check to make sure you have enough proteins, healthy fats, and high-fiber foods on hand, or add them to your grocery list.

☐ Prep the meals or foods that make sense to make over the weekend. Once you've completed your Preview, it will be easier to decide what needs to be prepped.

☐ Track your progress.

Track Your Progress

I suggest planning your meals out for the week here and coming back to add in your observations, but if you prefer, you can add them after you've already eaten them.

DAY	BREAKFAST	LUNCH	DINNER	SNACK	OBSERVATIONS (hunger levels, likes/dislikes)
Day 1					
Day 2					
Day 3					
Day 4					
Day 5					
Day 6					
Day 7					

Review Week Two

How many days did I stick to my new micro habit?

1 2 3 4 5 6 7

How many days was I able to continue with last week's micro habit as well?

1 2 3 4 5 6 7

How many days did I sleep seven or more hours?

1 2 3 4 5 6 7

How many days was I able to last at least four hours between meals?

1 2 3 4 5 6 7

How were my confidence levels this week?

Low   Average   High

How were my energy levels?

Low   Average   High

How were my stress levels?

Low   Average   High

Did I experience any digestive issues or bloating this week? ☐ Yes ☐ No

Notes:

Did I experience cravings or hangriness this week? ☐ Yes ☐ No

Notes:

What went well this week? What am I proud of?

What was a struggle?

_____

_____

_____

_____

_____

_____

_____

_____

_____

_____

_____

_____

Changes I'll make for next week:

_____

_____

_____

_____

_____

_____

_____

_____

_____

_____

_____

_____

_____

Week Three

MICRO HABIT: *Take a 20-minute power walk*

Why it matters: Zone 2 cardio is any kind of exercise where you are using 60–70 percent of your max heart rate. You'll know you're in zone 2 if you can maintain a conversation while having to pause on occasion to take a breath. Zone 2 cardio makes it easier for the body to burn fat for energy instead of always relying on carbohydrates.

While there is an endless parade of zone 2 activities you can get into, the one I love to recommend is the power walk. It is truly one of the most underrated tools for fat loss with a very low barrier to entry. You can even easily habit stack by taking your power walk after a meal to take advantage of the blood-sugar-lowering benefits.

For this week, I suggest just focusing on getting those 20 minutes of power walking in each day. Other zone 2 activities include biking, swimming, cleaning, or doing yard work. Just remember that in order to enter zone 2, you are still able to hold a conversation, but you have to pause on occasion to take a breath.

Ways to Power-Up Your Power Walks:

☐ Do a power walk on as flat a course as you can—a track is a great option.
☐ Try power walking up and down hills.
☐ Do the same walk three days in a row. Do you notice any difference in how it feels from day one to day three?
☐ Try your walk in the morning, at midday, and in the evening. Which gives you the greatest energy boost?

Additional Zone 2 Cardio Options to Try:

☐ biking (outside or stationary)
☐ swimming
☐ rowing (outside or erg machine)
☐ elliptical machine
☐ doing yard work
☐ cleaning

Preview Week Three

What's happening this week:

_____

_____

_____

_____

_____

_____

_____

Do a little brain dump of everything you've got going on this week. Dinners out, lunch meetings, soccer practice, date nights, meetings. Look at your calendar and lay it all out.

How to navigate obstacles:

_____

_____

_____

_____

_____

_____

_____

How will three soccer practices this week impact dinner? Your walks? How about the lunch meetings? Rushed mornings?

For example, you'd like to do your walks after work, but that will be impossible on nights you have events in the early evening. You plan your walks on your lunch break or schedule some walking meetings.

Checklist:

☐ Pull out your calendar and see where you can fit a 20-minute walk into your schedule. Schedule these walks in your calendar like you would a meeting.

☐ Do you need to bring walking shoes to work with you?

☐ Continue planning out breakfasts, lunches, and dinners for the week.

☐ Check to make sure you have enough proteins, healthy fats, and high-fiber foods on hand, or add them to your grocery list.

☐ Meal prep the meals or foods that make sense to meal prep over the weekend.

☐ Track your progress.

Track Your Progress

DAY	ACTIVITY + NUMBER OF MINUTES
Day 1	
Day 2	
Day 3	
Day 4	
Day 5	
Day 6	
Day 7	

Review Week Three

How many days did I stick
to my new micro habit?

1   2   3   4   5   6   7

How many days was I able to continue with
the previous weeks' micro habits as well?

1   2   3   4   5   6   7

How many days did I sleep
seven or more hours?

1   2   3   4   5   6   7

How many days was I able to last at
least four hours between meals?

1   2   3   4   5   6   7

How were my confidence
levels this week?

Low   Average   High

How were my energy levels?

Low   Average   High

How were my stress levels?

Low   Average   High

Did I experience any digestive issues
or bloating this week? ☐ Yes ☐ No

Notes:

Did I experience cravings or
hangriness this week? ☐ Yes ☐ No

Notes:

What went well this week? What am I proud of?

_____

_____

_____

_____

_____

_____

_____

_____

What was a struggle?

Changes I'll make for next week:

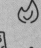

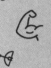
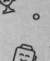

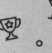

Week Four

MICRO HABIT: *Eat the right amount of carbs for your body*

Why it matters: You now know that eating carbs triggers an insulin response so that your cells can turn sugar into energy. If you eat more carbs than your body can immediately burn, the body will release a large amount of insulin, which limits the body's ability to burn fat. This also causes blood sugar spikes, which mean increased hunger and cravings.

But we need carbohydrates for energy, balanced hormones, and to build muscle! So how many carbs do you actually *need*? The amount depends on your age, level of physical activity, and various health conditions.

In the Metabolism Makeover method, we count the carbohydrates only in *starchy carbs*, like bread, rice, pasta, and potatoes, and not the carbohydrates you find in dairy, nuts, fruits, and nonstarchy vegetables. A key component to the Metabolism Makeover method is learning to eat the right amount of food to support your metabolism without tracking everything that goes into your mouth. This is a way to keep carbs in check without tracking your intake.

Below are some guidelines to get you started.

> » *First, use the chart on the next page to determine how many starchy carb servings your body needs each day.*

How to measure a serving size: One serving of starchy carbs is about 30–40 grams of carbs. So for example, ¾ cup of brown rice is 37 grams of carbs, which means it's one serving of starchy carbs. As for mashed potatoes, ½ cup is 19 grams of carbs, so you should bump up the serving to 1 cup. And then 1½ cups of pasta is 63 grams of carbs, so you can reduce to ¾ cup.

LIFE SITUATION	STARCHY CARB SERVINGS PER DAY
Strength training less than three times per week	one serving
Strength training more than three to four times per week	two servings
Blood-sugar-control issues (PCOS, insulin resistance, type 2 diabetes)	one serving
Perimenopause or menopause	one serving
Uncontrolled hypothyroidism, HPA axis dysfunction, or adrenal insufficiency diagnosis	three servings
Athletes, pregnant and breastfeeding women	three or more servings
For every two hours of moderate intensity cardio	one additional serving
For every one hour of high-intensity cardio	one additional serving

So for example, if you strength train four times per week, you would eat two servings of starchy carbs every day of the week. This might look like rice with your lunch and potatoes with dinner.

> » *Then, keep an eye on the following symptoms. If you experience any of the following, it's time to add an additional serving of starchy carbs:*

- ☐ **You are not progressing in your workouts.** You notice you're unable to increase the amount of weight you are lifting, and you feel depleted during the workouts.
- ☐ **Workout recovery is slow.** You're very sore and tired for at least a day after a workout.
- ☐ **Increased cravings**, especially in the evenings, even though you know you're eating PHFF all day.

> ### *Here are some good examples of starchy carbs:*
>
> - ☐ beans
> - ☐ beets
> - ☐ farro
> - ☐ lentils
> - ☐ oatmeal
> - ☐ peas
> - ☐ potatoes and sweet potatoes
>
> - ☐ high-fiber, whole-grain crackers (at least 3 grams of fiber per serving)
> - ☐ lentil or chickpea pasta
> - ☐ white, brown, or wild rice
> - ☐ quinoa
> - ☐ sourdough, whole-grain, or sprouted bread

Think about a typical day, and list the starchy carbs you're eating at each meal. Do your best to estimate how much you're eating as well.

Breakfast:

_____

_____

_____

_____

Dinner:

_____

_____

_____

_____

Lunch:

_____

_____

_____

_____

Snack:

_____

_____

_____

_____

On average, how many servings of starchy carbs are you eating each day? As a reminder, a serving is 30–40 grams of carbs, and we are including only starches and not the carbs in dairy, nuts, fruits, and nonstarchy vegetables.

_____

Based on what you've learned, do you need to increase or decrease the number of starchy carbs you're eating per day? Do you need to increase or decrease your serving sizes?

_____

Turn back to the lunch and dinner charts from week 2. Keep using those as your guide, but add starchy carbs from the lists below depending on how many you're eating each day.

LUNCH	DINNER
STARCHY CARBS (30–40 G)	**STARCHY CARBS (30–40 G)**
• ¼ cup uncooked or ⅔ cup cooked rice (white, brown, wild) • 2 servings crackers • 2 pieces whole-grain, sprouted, or sourdough bread • 2 oz lentil or chickpea pasta • ¾ cup baby red potatoes • ⅔ cup quinoa • ¼ cup uncooked or ¾ cup cooked lentils • ¾ cup chickpeas • 2 small tortillas	• 1 cup cooked corn • 1¼ cups cooked peas • ¼ cup uncooked or ⅔ cup cooked rice (white, brown, wild) • 2 small tortillas • ¼ cup uncooked or ¾ cup cooked lentils • 2 pieces whole-grain, sprouted, or sourdough bread • 2 oz dry lentil or chickpea pasta • ¾ cup baby red potatoes • ¼ cup uncooked or ⅔ cup cooked quinoa

Preview Week Four

What's happening this week:

_____

_____

_____

_____

_____

_____

How to navigate obstacles:

_____

_____

_____

_____

_____

_____

_____

_____

Checklist:

- ☐ Continue to plan out lunches and dinners for the week using the chart on page 101, but this time make sure you're eating the right amount of starchy carbs for your body.
- ☐ Check to make sure you have enough whole-food carbs on hand, and if not, add them to your grocery list.
- ☐ Meal prep over the weekend. How much you'll prep will vary based on how many starchy carbs you'll be eating.
- ☐ Schedule your walks.
- ☐ Track your progress.

Track Your Progress

Record the starchy carbs you eat and how many servings this week in the following chart.

DAY	STARCHY CARBS + SERVINGS	REFLECT ON ANY CHANGES IN ENERGY LEVELS, SATISFACTION/ FULLNESS, AND CRAVINGS
Day 1		
Day 2		
Day 3		
Day 4		
Day 5		
Day 6		
Day 7		

Review Week Four

How many days did I stick
to my new micro habit?

⭐ 1 ⭐ 2 ⭐ 3 ⭐ 4 ⭐ 5 ⭐ 6 ⭐ 7

How many days was I able to continue with
the previous weeks' micro habits as well?

⭐ 1 ⭐ 2 ⭐ 3 ⭐ 4 ⭐ 5 ⭐ 6 ⭐ 7

How many days did I sleep
seven or more hours?

⭐ 1 ⭐ 2 ⭐ 3 ⭐ 4 ⭐ 5 ⭐ 6 ⭐ 7

How many days was I able to last at
least four hours between meals?

⭐ 1 ⭐ 2 ⭐ 3 ⭐ 4 ⭐ 5 ⭐ 6 ⭐ 7

How were my confidence
levels this week?

Low   Average   High

How were my energy levels?

Low   Average   High

How were my stress levels?

Low   Average   High

Did I experience any digestive issues
or bloating this week? ☐ Yes ☐ No

Notes:

Did I experience cravings or
hangriness this week? ☐ Yes ☐ No

Notes:

What went well this week? What am I proud of?

_____
_____
_____
_____
_____
_____
_____
_____

What was a struggle?

Changes I'll make for next week:

Go back to page 71 and complete your Metabolic Movers assessment.

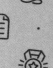

PART FOUR

Your Road Map for the Rest of the Year

At this point, you've spent some time practicing all five elements of YOU. You crafted your YOU statements and confronted your limiting beliefs. You learned about habits that move the metabolic needle, spent four weeks focused on building those habits, and used the Weekly Review/Preview to help you gain self-awareness around those habits.

The purpose of this past month was to help you really hit the ground running so that you could build momentum going into the rest of the year. This is what the rest of your year will now look like:

1. **You will choose one or two micro habits at a time to focus on.** You will not stack another micro habit until you feel solid in what you're currently working on. That could look like only adding one new micro habit every two, four, or even six weeks. This means that you might not incorporate all the micro habits until year two—and that's perfectly fine (and normal)!

2. **You will complete a Weekly Review/Preview just as you did during your first four weeks.** You will notice it looks slightly different as it will not be customized to a particular micro habit. This is because from here on out, you will be choosing which micro habit to work on week to week. As a reminder, this process is

incredibly important to keep up with as it helps inform you on how you are doing with implementing your habits and if adjustments need to be made.

The following is a master list of all the micro habits, organized by the pillars of the Metabolic Ecosystem, so you can choose your own micro habit adventure.

MASTER LIST OF MICRO HABITS

Blood sugar

- ☑ *Eat 30 grams of protein at breakfast.* Studies show a high-protein breakfast reduces calorie intake throughout the day. Plus, 30 grams of protein = muscle protein synthesis.
- ☑ *Eat PHFF at every meal.* The combination of protein, fat, and fiber at mealtime is the simplest way to keep blood sugar steady after meals.
- ☑ *Eat the right amount of carbs for your body.* Eating too many carbs is associated with blood sugar spikes, cravings, and excess fat storage. Eating too few carbs is associated with low energy levels, the inability to put on muscle, and increased stress in the body.
- ☐ *Hit your protein goal.* Protein is the best macronutrient to specifically target because it's supporting muscle, which is our metabolic money. Protein is the most satiating macronutrient.
- ☐ *Track your fiber intake.* The goal here is to make sure you're hitting at least 25 grams of fiber each day. Fiber is a powerful blood sugar controller, feeds healthy gut bacteria, and turns off hunger hormones.
- ☐ *Meal prep your most challenging meal.* This will help you hit PHFF goals and cut down on takeout or skipping meals, which lead to overeating. I've found it's much easier to hit protein goals when you meal prep.
- ☐ *Have PHFF lunches prepped and ready to go.* Same as above!
- ☐ *Have a smoothie for breakfast.* It's quick and easy to pack with PHFF and micronutrients. See the suggestions on page 87 to get you started.

☐ ***Track your fat intake.*** The goal here is to ensure you're eating no more than 30 grams at mealtimes, eating at least 60 grams per day, and staying under 100 grams per day.

☐ ***Prep two proteins per week.*** Protein tends to be the hardest macro-nutrient to hit if you're not prepared. This can include meal prep or simply making sure you have two types of premade proteins on hand for quick, easy, last-minute meals.

Muscle

☐ ***Strength train twice per week.*** Strength training twice per week is enough to trigger muscle growth, especially if you are a beginner. I recommend two full-body workouts.

☐ ***Strength train three times per week.*** Optimal workout frequency is less about the number of days and more about the number of sets worked out for each muscle group. For a typical workout with three to four sets per muscle group, a three-day workout split works well for both beginner and advanced weightlifters. I recommend three full-body workouts.

☐ ***Strength train four times per week.*** For advanced lifters, four strength sessions per week can increase the number of sets worked out for each muscle group. I recommend two upper body and two lower body workouts (instead of full-body workouts every time) so that you can have plenty of time to recover between muscle groups.

☐ ***Lay out workout clothes before going to bed.*** This can both serve as a reminder to work out as well as help remove the friction of having to pick out workout clothes in the morning.

☐ ***Bring workout clothes to work with you and change into them at the end of the day.*** You don't *have* to go to the gym or do your home workout just because you put your workout clothes on, but it's still going to signal to your brain that it's time to work out.

☐ ***Schedule workouts in your calendar.*** If you schedule workouts like a meeting, you'll treat them like one!

Movement

- [x] **Take a 20-minute power walk.** Getting in zone 2 for 20 minutes every day makes it easier for the body to burn fat for energy instead of always relying on carbohydrates.
- [ ] **Create and hit a step goal.** Find the average number of steps you take in a day and increase that by 1,000 steps. For example, if you typically get 4,000 steps a day, increase that to 5,000. Once you have that down, push yourself to increase to 6,000, and so on.
- [ ] **Use a standing desk for 50 percent of the workday.** Standing significantly reduces post-meal blood sugar levels when compared to sitting.
- [ ] **Take a 10–20-minute walk after each meal.** Blood sugar levels hit a peak within 90 minutes of a meal, and a post-meal walk reduces blood sugar spikes.
- [ ] **Do 10 minutes of yoga, stretching, or mobility work once a day.** We often think of movement as something that helps us in the *now*: it burns more calories, steadies blood sugar, and increases metabolic flexibility. But stretching and mobility work can help us continue to be able to move freely as we age.

Sleep

- [ ] **Maintain a consistent bedtime.** Pick a bedtime that works for your schedule this week, and go to sleep within 30 minutes of that time each night.
- [ ] **Stop using screens at least 30 minutes before bed.** Blue light from screens disrupts the release of our sleepy hormone, melatonin.
- [ ] **Wear amber-colored, blue-light blockers at least two hours before bedtime.** Cutting down on any form of blue light in the hours before bedtime will encourage more melatonin production.
- [ ] **Eliminate alcohol during the week, minimum.** Alcohol acts on your calming neurotransmitter, GABA, causing you to wake up multiple times in the night without realizing it. It also disrupts REM sleep, a critical repair time for the body and brain.

- ☐ ***Avoid caffeine 8–10 hours before bed.*** Everyone has a different caffeine tolerance, but you can start scaling back by 15 minutes a day until you settle on a time that doesn't seem to affect your sleep.
- ☐ ***Begin turning off extra lights around 6:00 p.m.*** This will help with the release of sleep-promoting hormones.
- ☐ ***Get 10 minutes of morning light outside.*** Morning sunlight triggers a melatonin release around 14 hours later. This is especially helpful if you are not getting tired early enough in the evening.

Stress

- ☐ ***Schedule stress management.*** Our high-stress lives require a daily hygiene practice around managing stress. It's just as important as scheduling a workout, meal prep, or anything else that takes high priority.
- ☐ ***Choose three things to do that bring you joy each day.*** These should bring you joy both during and after the activity (if you feel joy after a workout because it's over, it doesn't count!). It can be as small as five minutes alone with a cup of coffee.
- ☐ ***Do gratitude journaling before bed.*** Gratitude journaling is simple: just write down a list of things you are grateful for. To begin, you might just jot down three to five things that can be as small as "the beautiful clouds in the sky" or "the way my cat snuggled with me."
- ☐ ***Spend at least 20 minutes outside.*** The benefits of being outside, in nature if possible, are endless.
- ☐ ***Freewrite every day for 10 minutes.*** Freewriting is exactly what it sounds like: no prompts, no grammar or spelling police, no stopping. Just set a timer and let anything and everything flow out of your pen.
- ☐ ***Do a time and energy audit.*** What are you actually spending your time on? What can you eliminate from your to-do list to give yourself back some precious time (so you can use it for some of these micro habits)? Pull back your people-pleasing tendencies and get ruthless about your time.
- ☐ ***Start a breath work practice.*** Breath work is any kind of practice where you control your breath. A simple one is box breath: breathe in

for four seconds, hold for four, breathe out for four, hold for four, and repeat. Wim Hof Method or SOMA Breath are other methods you can find on YouTube. Try a different practice each day, or do the same one the whole week, and see how it goes.

☐ *Start an affirmation practice.* Affirmations are any positive statements that resonate with you. Record a few that light you up on your phone, and listen to them every morning.

☐ *Do a social media detox.* Every time you have a negative emotion when looking at a social media post—whether it's because the post itself is negative or because you're comparing your life or your body to someone else's—it creates a stress response. Get rid of that unnecessary stress by limiting how often you go on social media or taking a break altogether.

☐ *Delete news apps from your phone.* Same as above!

Gut health

☐ *Chew each bite of food 20–30 times.* Indigestion and bloating can have several culprits, but one may be that you're simply not chewing your food to a consistency that allows for proper digestion. Food should have the consistency of applesauce before swallowing.

☐ *Add a daily mineral drink.* There are many mineral and electrolyte drink brands on the market now, and while we often think of them as ways to better hydrate, minerals also have a big impact on our gut! Potassium, sodium, and magnesium are the most important to start with.

☐ *Include two to three different fermented foods per day.* These contain healthy bacteria that populate the gut and can include sauerkraut, kimchi, raw pickles, kombucha, raw dairy products, homemade sourdough bread or crackers, miso, and tempeh.

☐ *Eat a minimum of five different plants (fruits, vegetables, nuts, legumes, etc.) per day.* Plants contain prebiotic fiber, and prebiotic fiber feeds healthy bacteria. Getting a variety of prebiotics in the diet has been shown to have the greatest impact on gut health.

TIPS TO HELP YOU MAP OUT YOUR YEAR

1. Go back to the Create Your Vision activity on page 45. What gaps do you need to fill to make your vision a reality?

2. Consider the time of year and your current season of life. For example, a 20-minute walk may not be a top choice in the dead of winter in the northeastern United States, and eight hours of sleep is probably not realistic if you're four months postpartum. Set yourself up for success by choosing micro habits that feel like a challenge but are still totally doable.

3. Give yourself a head start by mapping out your entire year at once (knowing you'll likely make edits as you go) or by tackling it one month at a time. This will very much depend on how you like to plan and organize your life, but either of these is easier than going week by week.

4. Once you know which micro habit you're going to start with, review the Metabolic Ecosystem pillar it correlates to in part 1 starting on page 2.

If you're still unsure of where to start, use the QR code below to take you to the Metabolic Ecosystem quiz to see which pillars you're falling short on and start there.

SAMPLE ROAD MAPS

You still might be wondering exactly how to go about choosing your micro habits throughout the year. While there's no right or wrong way to do this, I suggest focusing on what you feel is easy enough to implement *now* while also stretching yourself into that version of YOU that you defined in the vision section. To help bring this to life, I'm going to introduce you to Audrey and Joyce, and we'll take a look at how each of them handles the year.

> *Audrey*

Audrey struggles with sleep deprivation and stress. It's hard for her to get in workouts and nail her nutrition because she feels like she's burning the candle at both ends. She's exhausted and struggles with putting herself first. After gaining some momentum with her diet and daily walks in the Four-Week Jump Start, Audrey has a clear sense of the direction she wants to go in the rest of the year.

But before I walk you through her sample road map, let's take a look at Audrey's thought process around why she chose the micro habits she chose to work on right off the bat, as well as her thinking (and progress!) as the year unfolds.

First, Audrey decides she wants to tackle sleep micro habits for two solid months to get her exhaustion under control.

As she begins to get more sleep and feel more rested, she notices her stress starts to decrease without actually incorporating any stress-management practices! Because she now has more energy, she decides to start strength training and then work on one of her more difficult meals to stick to consistently—lunch.

By the sixth month, while she is feeling better due to better sleep, she knows she still has a lot of work to do in the stress-management department, so she commits to 10 minutes of breath work per day. Audrey also wants to push herself to see more muscle gains in the gym. She bumps her strength-training workouts to three times a week and really dials in on her protein goals.

At this point, Audrey is feeling more confident and less stressed than she has in years, so she begins addressing her people-pleasing tendencies by auditing her energy and time every week. She also decides to get off the treadmill, where she's been doing her daily walks, and get outside for sunlight and fresh air.

About nine months in, Audrey's weight loss stalls, and she decides to check her fat intake. She realizes she's been overdoing the fat, consciously cuts back, and starts seeing results again. At this point, Audrey's focus is less about correcting bad habits; instead, she is now focused only on enhancing the foundation she's already set throughout the year by including more gut-friendly foods in her diet.

Week 1–4: Blood Sugar

☐ Eat 30 grams of protein at breakfast.

☐ Eat PHFF at every meal.

☐ Take a 20-minute power walk.

☐ Eat the right amount of carbs for your body.

Week 5–8: Sleep

☐ Wear amber-colored, blue-light blockers at least two hours before bedtime.

☐ Get 10 minutes of morning light outside.

Week 9–12: Sleep

☐ Stop using screens at least 30 minutes before bed.

☐ Eliminate alcohol during the week, minimum.

Week 13–16: Muscle

☐ Strength train twice per week.

Week 17–20: PHFF

☐ Have PHFF lunches prepped and ready to go.

Week 21–24: Stress

☐ Start a breath work practice. Do 10 minutes a day.

Week 21–24: Blood Sugar

☐ Hit your protein goal.

Week 25–28: Muscle

☐ Strength train three times per week.

Week 29–32: Stress

☐ Do a time and energy audit.

☐ Spend at least 20 minutes outside.

Week 33–36: PHFF

☐ Track your fat intake.

Week 37–40: Gut Health

☐ Eat a minimum of five different plants (fruits, vegetables, nuts, legumes, etc.) per day.

Week 41–44: Gut Health

☐ Add a daily mineral drink.

Week 45–48: Gut Health

☐ Include two to three different fermented foods per day.

Week 49–52: PHFF

☐ Track your fiber intake.

Joyce

Joyce has been struggling with weight gain for a few years now. She's been a yo-yo-dieting-and-cardio bunny for as long as she can remember, and it feels like it's finally catching up with her.

After completely obliterating every belief she has ever had about weight loss during the Four-Week Jump Start, Joyce is starting to feel really, *really* good. It was a tough learning curve to switch from counting calories to building a plate based on her blood sugar, but her cravings and binge-eating episodes have almost completely vanished.

She decided to throw out her beliefs about daily cardio, too, and replace three of her runs with strength training. Not only did she begin to feel stronger and more confident within those four weeks, but she also found she had more energy and felt less inflamed. You could say Joyce is now a believer.

She upped her strength to four times per week, but she started to feel weak in her workouts. She revisited how many carbs she is supposed to be eating and realized she has been undereating. Joyce is used to undereating carbs from years of dieting, making this one tough for her to adjust to, so she decided to repeat this micro habit for a month.

She's also had gut issues for a long time, so she spent a month working on gut health. It doesn't seem like anything is working to improve her gut, but she's grateful for the knowledge she now has about her gut and decides it's time she makes an appointment with a functional gut specialist to address this.

At this point, Joyce's diet and exercise regimen has changed completely and is going well. She's steadily losing fat and gaining muscle. But now she wonders what all this stress-management stuff is about in relation to metabolism. As a long-term dieter, this is a new concept. She starts by unfollowing social media accounts that make her feel bad and starts adding more joy into her day. It feels so good that she spends eight solid weeks working on stress.

Because Joyce is so in tune with her body now, she is realizing alcohol makes her feel foggy and less rested the next day, so she eliminates her nightly glass of wine. Earlier this year, she had attempted to do the daily smoothies for an easy breakfast, but it didn't stick. Now she tries it out again because her new job requires her to come in earlier.

Joyce finishes out her year by perfecting her protein for muscle gains, adding in more walks because she's enjoying them over running, and adding in some nightly stretching for mobility and as a way to wind down.

Week 1–4: Blood Sugar

- ☐ Eat 30 grams of protein at breakfast.
- ☐ Eat PHFF at every meal.
- ☐ Take a 20-minute power walk.
- ☐ Eat the right amount of carbs for your body.

Week 5–8: Muscle

- ☐ Strength train three times per week.

Week 9–12: Muscle

- ☐ Strength train four times per week.

Week 13–16: PHFF

- ☐ Eat the right amount of carbs for your body.

Week 17–20: PHFF

- ☐ Track your fiber intake.
- ☐ Have a smoothie for breakfast.

Week 21–24: Gut Health

- ☐ Chew each bite of food 20–30 times.
- ☐ Add a daily mineral drink.

Week 25–28: Stress

- ☐ Do a social media detox.
- ☐ Choose three things to do that bring you joy each day.

Week 29–32: Stress

- ☐ Practice affirmations.

Week 33–36: Sleep

- ☐ Eliminate alcohol during the week, minimum.

Week 37–40: PHFF

- ☐ Have a smoothie for breakfast.

Week 41–44: PHFF

- ☐ Hit your protein goal.

Week 45-48: Movement

- ☐ Take a 10–20-minute walk after each meal.

Week 49–52: Movement

- ☐ Do 10 minutes of yoga, stretching, or mobility work once a day.

ACCOUNTABILITY GROUPS

I know what you're thinking: *I'm committed, but a year is a long time. Can I get any extra support?*

You bet! As a matter of fact, I recommend it. When I recently polled a thousand of my current clients to find out what they believed contributed to their success doing this method, one of the top three answers was the accountability and support they receive doing it in a group setting with like-minded people. (The other two answers were vision work and learning the science behind their metabolism.) You can join others in your metabolism makeover on my website at metabolismmakeover.co or by scanning the QR code below.

WHAT DO I DO WHEN . . . ?

At this point, you may be really excited to map out your year like Audrey and Joyce, but the reality is that your year will likely not play out exactly how you plan it. As a matter of fact, I'd be willing to bet your week usually doesn't play out exactly how you plan it!

For example: The office brings in donuts. A spontaneous date night pops up. You're in a situation where you have no control over your food choices. You skip a workout when plans change. Now what?

Choice #1: Go into "fuck-it mode," take a ride on the shame train, and start over on Monday.

Choice #2: Ask yourself, what's my next best choice?

The Next Best Choice Framework is a deliberate process you can walk through any time you find yourself in a situation where you are consciously choosing to stay on track or deviate from the track. When you start to use the Next Best Choice Framework, you'll likely have to consciously walk through each step deliberately. But eventually, this will become a subconscious practice that you won't even have to think about! This right here is your ticket to freedom. Let's take a look:

Next Best Choice: Version #1

Step 1: Pause. When you find yourself in a situation where there is something that you want to eat that doesn't balance your blood sugar, consciously take a beat.

Step 2: Walk through your options. What will happen and how will you feel if you decide to eat this food? How will it be metabolized in your body? How will it make you feel in the moment? In an hour? How will you feel emotionally?

Step 3: Make a decision, and then make a plan (if needed). If you decide to eat the food, that's okay! Just ask yourself, *What is the next best choice that I can make after eating this food?* This might be choosing what other foods to eat *with* the food you chose, or it might be planning how you'll handle a potential blood sugar crash later.

And when you find yourself in a situation where you've already eaten the donut or the entire bowl of chips and queso, this framework still applies! It just looks a bit different:

Next Best Choice: Version #2

Step 1: Pause. Take a beat, come back to the present moment, and remind yourself that *you did not fail, because you cannot fail at this.*

Step 2: Walk through what happens next. How will this food be metabolized? Are you going to experience a blood sugar crash later? If so, what can you do next?

Step 3: Decide what happens next. Go for a walk to stabilize your blood sugar, or get in a resistance workout so that your muscle glycogen can soak up some of those wonderful carbs for strength building. Decide on your next blood-sugar-balancing meal. Drink water. Breathe. Move on! You got this.

You may not realize how often you deviate from the track between weekends, nights out, and travel, and if you're not utilizing the Next Best Choice Framework, it could be seriously impacting your ability to see progress.

Road Map Reflection and Activity

To prepare for when you get off track during the following year, take the following steps:

Step 1: Take a moment and break down your year. Approximately how many days include weekends, travel, holidays, date nights, or any other off-the-track moments? This will be an estimate, of course, but do your best.

January _____   July _____

February _____   August _____

March _____   September _____

April _____   October _____

May _____   November _____

June _____   December _____

What percentage of your year is off the track?

_____ off-the-track days / 365 = _____ % off the track

Step 2: What does a typical day look like if you go off the track?

_____

_____

_____

_____

_____

_____

_____

_____

_____

_____

_____

_____

_____

_____

_____

Step 3: What if you never threw yourself off the track or started over on a Monday? Instead, you can choose consistency over perfection. What would be different about your life today? What would be different about your body?

There's no right or wrong way to choose **which micro habits** *to focus on. Start with what you feel is* **easy enough to implement now** *while also* **stretching** *yourself into that version of* **YOU** *that you defined earlier.*

WEEKLY CHECK-INS: WEEKS FIVE THROUGH FIFTY-TWO

You've already had some practice reviewing your previous week and previewing your upcoming week. You will continue this process each week for the rest of the year, and it should take you anywhere from 10 to 30 minutes. Rest assured, the amount of time it's going to give back to you—in the short term and the long term—is worth every minute.

Here's how this weekly process will work:

First, choose a day to complete your Review/Preview. Most readers opt to complete this exercise on a Saturday or Sunday. When it's your designated day, you will:

1. **Review your previous week.** The purpose of this review is to look at what went well and what didn't and then use that information to create positive change in your upcoming week.
2. **Preview your upcoming week.** Choose a micro habit to work on, then make plans and arrange your schedule in a way that supports consistency with that habit as well as any previous habits you've implemented.

REVIEW PREVIOUS WEEK

DATE:

Rate yourself from 1 (it was a struggle) to 5 (100% full success!).

Microhabit	1 2 3 (4) 5	Cravings / Feeling hangry	1 2 3 (4) 5
4 hours between meals	1 2 3 4 (5)	Confidence	1 2 3 (4) 5
Energy levels	1 2 (3) 4 5	Stress levels	1 2 (3) 4 5
Digestion/Bloating	1 2 3 4 (5)	Sleep	1 2 (3) 4 5

What went well this week? What am I proud of? *My nutrition was on point!*

What was a struggle? *It was a stressful week, which impacted my sleep + energy levels.*

Changes I'll make for next week: *I will really prioritize sleep + turn my phone off to reduce stress.*

PREVIEW UPCOMING WEEK

Micro habit of the week: *Phone off by 9 pm*

What's happening this week: *Happy hour at 4pm on Wednesday, gymnastics at 4:30pm on Thursday, lunch meeting on Friday, dinner + drinks at 7pm on Saturday.*

How to navigate any obstacles to habits: *Happy hour + gymnastics will disrupt getting my 2nd workout in, so I'll make up for it over the weekend. Dinner + drinks may disrupt my sleep on Sunday, but I'm going to stick to 1 drink to minimize sleep disruptions.*

REVIEW PREVIOUS WEEK

DATE:

Transfer some of your week 4 review notes from page 104 here to get started!

Rate yourself from 1 (it was a struggle) to 5 (100% full success!).

Micro habit	1 2 3 4 5	Cravings / Feeling hangry	1 2 3 4 5
4 hours between meals	1 2 3 4 5	Confidence	1 2 3 4 5
Energy levels	1 2 3 4 5	Stress levels	1 2 3 4 5
Digestion/Bloating	1 2 3 4 5	Sleep	1 2 3 4 5

What went well this week? What am I proud of? _____
_____
_____

What was a struggle? _____
_____
_____

Changes I'll make for next week: _____
_____
_____
_____

PREVIEW UPCOMING WEEK

Micro habit of the week: _____

What's happening this week: _____
_____
_____
_____

How to navigate any obstacles to habits: _____
_____
_____
_____
_____

REVIEW PREVIOUS WEEK

DATE:

Rate yourself from 1 (it was a struggle) to 5 (100% full success!).

Micro habit	1 2 3 4 5	Cravings / Feeling hangry	1 2 3 4 5
4 hours between meals	1 2 3 4 5	Confidence	1 2 3 4 5
Energy levels	1 2 3 4 5	Stress levels	1 2 3 4 5
Digestion/Bloating	1 2 3 4 5	Sleep	1 2 3 4 5

What went well this week? What am I proud of?

What was a struggle?

Changes I'll make for next week:

PREVIEW UPCOMING WEEK

Micro habit of the week:

What's happening this week:

How to navigate any obstacles to habits:

REVIEW PREVIOUS WEEK

DATE:

Rate yourself from 1 (it was a struggle) to 5 (100% full success!).

Micro habit	1 2 3 4 5	Cravings / Feeling hangry	1 2 3 4 5
4 hours between meals	1 2 3 4 5	Confidence	1 2 3 4 5
Energy levels	1 2 3 4 5	Stress levels	1 2 3 4 5
Digestion/Bloating	1 2 3 4 5	Sleep	1 2 3 4 5

What went well this week? What am I proud of?

_____

_____

What was a struggle?

_____

_____

Changes I'll make for next week:

_____

_____

_____

PREVIEW UPCOMING WEEK

Micro habit of the week: _____

What's happening this week: _____

_____

_____

How to navigate any obstacles to habits: _____

_____

_____

_____

REVIEW PREVIOUS WEEK

DATE:

Rate yourself from 1 (it was a struggle) to 5 (100% full success!).

Micro habit	1 2 3 4 5	Cravings / Feeling hangry	1 2 3 4 5
4 hours between meals	1 2 3 4 5	Confidence	1 2 3 4 5
Energy levels	1 2 3 4 5	Stress levels	1 2 3 4 5
Digestion/Bloating	1 2 3 4 5	Sleep	1 2 3 4 5

What went well this week? What am I proud of?

_____

_____

_____

What was a struggle?

_____

_____

_____

Changes I'll make for next week:

_____

_____

_____

PREVIEW UPCOMING WEEK

Micro habit of the week: _____

What's happening this week: _____

_____

_____

_____

How to navigate any obstacles to habits: _____

_____

_____

_____

REVIEW PREVIOUS WEEK

DATE:

Rate yourself from 1 (it was a struggle) to 5 (100% full success!).

Micro habit	1 2 3 4 5	Cravings / Feeling hangry	1 2 3 4 5
4 hours between meals	1 2 3 4 5	Confidence	1 2 3 4 5
Energy levels	1 2 3 4 5	Stress levels	1 2 3 4 5
Digestion/Bloating	1 2 3 4 5	Sleep	1 2 3 4 5

What went well this week? What am I proud of? _____
_____
_____

What was a struggle? _____
_____
_____

Changes I'll make for next week: _____
_____
_____
_____

PREVIEW UPCOMING WEEK

Micro habit of the week: _____

What's happening this week: _____
_____
_____

How to navigate any obstacles to habits: _____
_____
_____
_____
_____

REVIEW PREVIOUS WEEK

DATE:

Rate yourself from 1 (it was a struggle) to 5 (100% full success!).

Micro habit	1 2 3 4 5	Cravings / Feeling hangry	1 2 3 4 5
4 hours between meals	1 2 3 4 5	Confidence	1 2 3 4 5
Energy levels	1 2 3 4 5	Stress levels	1 2 3 4 5
Digestion/Bloating	1 2 3 4 5	Sleep	1 2 3 4 5

What went well this week? What am I proud of?

_____

_____

What was a struggle?

_____

_____

Changes I'll make for next week: _____

_____

_____

PREVIEW UPCOMING WEEK

Micro habit of the week: _____

What's happening this week: _____

_____

_____

How to navigate any obstacles to habits: _____

_____

_____

_____

REVIEW PREVIOUS WEEK

DATE:

Rate yourself from 1 (it was a struggle) to 5 (100% full success!).

Micro habit	1 2 3 4 5	Cravings / Feeling hangry	1 2 3 4 5
4 hours between meals	1 2 3 4 5	Confidence	1 2 3 4 5
Energy levels	1 2 3 4 5	Stress levels	1 2 3 4 5
Digestion/Bloating	1 2 3 4 5	Sleep	1 2 3 4 5

What went well this week? What am I proud of? _____

_____

_____

What was a struggle? _____

_____

_____

Changes I'll make for next week: _____

_____

_____

_____

PREVIEW UPCOMING WEEK

Micro habit of the week: _____

What's happening this week: _____

_____

_____

_____

How to navigate any obstacles to habits: _____

_____

_____

_____

_____

REVIEW PREVIOUS WEEK

DATE:

Rate yourself from 1 (it was a struggle) to 5 (100% full success!).

Micro habit	1 2 3 4 5	Cravings / Feeling hangry	1 2 3 4 5
4 hours between meals	1 2 3 4 5	Confidence	1 2 3 4 5
Energy levels	1 2 3 4 5	Stress levels	1 2 3 4 5
Digestion/Bloating	1 2 3 4 5	Sleep	1 2 3 4 5

What went well this week? What am I proud of?

_____

_____

What was a struggle?

_____

_____

Changes I'll make for next week:

_____

_____

_____

PREVIEW UPCOMING WEEK

Micro habit of the week: _____

What's happening this week: _____

_____

_____

How to navigate any obstacles to habits: _____

_____

_____

_____

REVIEW PREVIOUS WEEK

DATE:

Rate yourself from 1 (it was a struggle) to 5 (100% full success!).

Micro habit	1 2 3 4 5	Cravings / Feeling hangry	1 2 3 4 5
4 hours between meals	1 2 3 4 5	Confidence	1 2 3 4 5
Energy levels	1 2 3 4 5	Stress levels	1 2 3 4 5
Digestion/Bloating	1 2 3 4 5	Sleep	1 2 3 4 5

What went well this week? What am I proud of? _____
_____
_____

What was a struggle? _____
_____
_____

Changes I'll make for next week: _____
_____
_____
_____

PREVIEW UPCOMING WEEK

Micro habit of the week: _____

What's happening this week: _____
_____
_____
_____

How to navigate any obstacles to habits: _____
_____
_____
_____
_____

REVIEW PREVIOUS WEEK

DATE:

Rate yourself from 1 (it was a struggle) to 5 (100% full success!).

Micro habit	1 2 3 4 5	Cravings / Feeling hangry	1 2 3 4 5
4 hours between meals	1 2 3 4 5	Confidence	1 2 3 4 5
Energy levels	1 2 3 4 5	Stress levels	1 2 3 4 5
Digestion/Bloating	1 2 3 4 5	Sleep	1 2 3 4 5

What went well this week? What am I proud of?

What was a struggle?

Changes I'll make for next week:

PREVIEW UPCOMING WEEK

Micro habit of the week:

What's happening this week:

How to navigate any obstacles to habits:

REVIEW PREVIOUS WEEK

DATE:

Rate yourself from 1 (it was a struggle) to 5 (100% full success!).

Micro habit	1 2 3 4 5	Cravings / Feeling hangry	1 2 3 4 5
4 hours between meals	1 2 3 4 5	Confidence	1 2 3 4 5
Energy levels	1 2 3 4 5	Stress levels	1 2 3 4 5
Digestion/Bloating	1 2 3 4 5	Sleep	1 2 3 4 5

What went well this week? What am I proud of? _____
_____
_____

What was a struggle? _____
_____
_____

Changes I'll make for next week: _____
_____
_____
_____

PREVIEW UPCOMING WEEK

Micro habit of the week: _____

What's happening this week: _____
_____
_____
_____

How to navigate any obstacles to habits: _____
_____
_____
_____
_____

REVIEW PREVIOUS WEEK

DATE:

Rate yourself from 1 (it was a struggle) to 5 (100% full success!).

Micro habit	1 2 3 4 5	Cravings / Feeling hangry	1 2 3 4 5
4 hours between meals	1 2 3 4 5	Confidence	1 2 3 4 5
Energy levels	1 2 3 4 5	Stress levels	1 2 3 4 5
Digestion/Bloating	1 2 3 4 5	Sleep	1 2 3 4 5

What went well this week? What am I proud of?

What was a struggle?

Changes I'll make for next week:

PREVIEW UPCOMING WEEK

Micro habit of the week:

What's happening this week:

How to navigate any obstacles to habits:

REVIEW PREVIOUS WEEK

DATE:

Rate yourself from 1 (it was a struggle) to 5 (100% full success!).

Micro habit	1 2 3 4 5	Cravings / Feeling hangry	1 2 3 4 5
4 hours between meals	1 2 3 4 5	Confidence	1 2 3 4 5
Energy levels	1 2 3 4 5	Stress levels	1 2 3 4 5
Digestion/Bloating	1 2 3 4 5	Sleep	1 2 3 4 5

What went well this week? What am I proud of? _____
_____
_____

What was a struggle? _____
_____
_____

Changes I'll make for next week: _____
_____
_____
_____

PREVIEW UPCOMING WEEK

Micro habit of the week: _____

What's happening this week: _____
_____
_____
_____

How to navigate any obstacles to habits: _____
_____
_____
_____

REVIEW PREVIOUS WEEK

DATE:

Rate yourself from 1 (it was a struggle) to 5 (100% full success!).

Micro habit	1 2 3 4 5	Cravings / Feeling hangry	1 2 3 4 5
4 hours between meals	1 2 3 4 5	Confidence	1 2 3 4 5
Energy levels	1 2 3 4 5	Stress levels	1 2 3 4 5
Digestion/Bloating	1 2 3 4 5	Sleep	1 2 3 4 5

What went well this week? What am I proud of?

What was a struggle?

Changes I'll make for next week:

PREVIEW UPCOMING WEEK

Micro habit of the week:

What's happening this week:

How to navigate any obstacles to habits:

REVIEW PREVIOUS WEEK

DATE:

Rate yourself from 1 (it was a struggle) to 5 (100% full success!).

Micro habit	1 2 3 4 5	Cravings / Feeling hangry	1 2 3 4 5
4 hours between meals	1 2 3 4 5	Confidence	1 2 3 4 5
Energy levels	1 2 3 4 5	Stress levels	1 2 3 4 5
Digestion/Bloating	1 2 3 4 5	Sleep	1 2 3 4 5

What went well this week? What am I proud of?

_____

_____

_____

What was a struggle?

_____

_____

_____

Changes I'll make for next week:

_____

_____

_____

_____

PREVIEW UPCOMING WEEK

Micro habit of the week:

_____

What's happening this week:

_____

_____

_____

_____

How to navigate any obstacles to habits:

_____

_____

_____

_____

_____

Rate yourself from 1 (it was a struggle) to 5 (100% full success!).

Micro habit	1 2 3 4 5	Cravings / Feeling hangry	1 2 3 4 5
4 hours between meals	1 2 3 4 5	Confidence	1 2 3 4 5
Energy levels	1 2 3 4 5	Stress levels	1 2 3 4 5
Digestion/Bloating	1 2 3 4 5	Sleep	1 2 3 4 5

What went well this week? What am I proud of?

What was a struggle?

Changes I'll make for next week:

PREVIEW UPCOMING WEEK

Micro habit of the week:

What's happening this week:

How to navigate any obstacles to habits:

REVIEW PREVIOUS WEEK

DATE:

Rate yourself from 1 (it was a struggle) to 5 (100% full success!).

Micro habit	1 2 3 4 5	Cravings / Feeling hangry	1 2 3 4 5
4 hours between meals	1 2 3 4 5	Confidence	1 2 3 4 5
Energy levels	1 2 3 4 5	Stress levels	1 2 3 4 5
Digestion/Bloating	1 2 3 4 5	Sleep	1 2 3 4 5

What went well this week? What am I proud of? _____

_____

_____

What was a struggle? _____

_____

_____

Changes I'll make for next week: _____

_____

_____

_____

PREVIEW UPCOMING WEEK

Micro habit of the week: _____

What's happening this week: _____

_____

_____

_____

How to navigate any obstacles to habits: _____

_____

_____

_____

REVIEW PREVIOUS WEEK

DATE:

Rate yourself from 1 (it was a struggle) to 5 (100% full success!).

Micro habit	1 2 3 4 5	Cravings / Feeling hangry	1 2 3 4 5
4 hours between meals	1 2 3 4 5	Confidence	1 2 3 4 5
Energy levels	1 2 3 4 5	Stress levels	1 2 3 4 5
Digestion/Bloating	1 2 3 4 5	Sleep	1 2 3 4 5

What went well this week? What am I proud of?

_____

_____

What was a struggle?

_____

_____

Changes I'll make for next week:

_____

_____

_____

PREVIEW UPCOMING WEEK

Micro habit of the week: _____

What's happening this week: _____

_____

_____

How to navigate any obstacles to habits: _____

_____

_____

_____

REVIEW PREVIOUS WEEK

DATE:

Rate yourself from 1 (it was a struggle) to 5 (100% full success!).

Micro habit	1 2 3 4 5	Cravings / Feeling hangry	1 2 3 4 5
4 hours between meals	1 2 3 4 5	Confidence	1 2 3 4 5
Energy levels	1 2 3 4 5	Stress levels	1 2 3 4 5
Digestion/Bloating	1 2 3 4 5	Sleep	1 2 3 4 5

What went well this week? What am I proud of?

What was a struggle?

Changes I'll make for next week:

PREVIEW UPCOMING WEEK

Micro habit of the week:

What's happening this week:

How to navigate any obstacles to habits:

REVIEW PREVIOUS WEEK

DATE:

Rate yourself from 1 (it was a struggle) to 5 (100% full success!).

Micro habit	1 2 3 4 5	Cravings / Feeling hangry	1 2 3 4 5
4 hours between meals	1 2 3 4 5	Confidence	1 2 3 4 5
Energy levels	1 2 3 4 5	Stress levels	1 2 3 4 5
Digestion/Bloating	1 2 3 4 5	Sleep	1 2 3 4 5

What went well this week? What am I proud of?

What was a struggle?

Changes I'll make for next week:

PREVIEW UPCOMING WEEK

Micro habit of the week:

What's happening this week:

How to navigate any obstacles to habits:

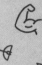
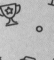

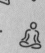

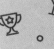

DATE:

Rate yourself from 1 (it was a struggle) to 5 (100% full success!).

Micro habit	1 2 3 4 5	Cravings / Feeling hangry	1 2 3 4 5
4 hours between meals	1 2 3 4 5	Confidence	1 2 3 4 5
Energy levels	1 2 3 4 5	Stress levels	1 2 3 4 5
Digestion/Bloating	1 2 3 4 5	Sleep	1 2 3 4 5

What went well this week? What am I proud of? _____

_____

_____

What was a struggle? _____

_____

_____

Changes I'll make for next week: _____

_____

_____

_____

PREVIEW UPCOMING WEEK

Micro habit of the week: _____

What's happening this week: _____

_____

_____

How to navigate any obstacles to habits: _____

_____

_____

_____

_____

REVIEW PREVIOUS WEEK

DATE:

Rate yourself from 1 (it was a struggle) to 5 (100% full success!).

Micro habit	1 2 3 4 5	Cravings / Feeling hangry	1 2 3 4 5
4 hours between meals	1 2 3 4 5	Confidence	1 2 3 4 5
Energy levels	1 2 3 4 5	Stress levels	1 2 3 4 5
Digestion/Bloating	1 2 3 4 5	Sleep	1 2 3 4 5

What went well this week? What am I proud of?

What was a struggle?

Changes I'll make for next week:

PREVIEW UPCOMING WEEK

Micro habit of the week:

What's happening this week:

How to navigate any obstacles to habits:

REVIEW PREVIOUS WEEK

DATE:

Rate yourself from 1 (it was a struggle) to 5 (100% full success!).

Micro habit	1 2 3 4 5	Cravings / Feeling hangry	1 2 3 4 5
4 hours between meals	1 2 3 4 5	Confidence	1 2 3 4 5
Energy levels	1 2 3 4 5	Stress levels	1 2 3 4 5
Digestion/Bloating	1 2 3 4 5	Sleep	1 2 3 4 5

What went well this week? What am I proud of?

_____

_____

_____

What was a struggle?

_____

_____

_____

Changes I'll make for next week:

_____

_____

_____

_____

PREVIEW UPCOMING WEEK

Micro habit of the week: _____

What's happening this week: _____

_____

_____

_____

How to navigate any obstacles to habits: _____

_____

_____

_____

_____

REVIEW PREVIOUS WEEK

DATE:

Rate yourself from 1 (it was a struggle) to 5 (100% full success!).

Micro habit	1 2 3 4 5	Cravings / Feeling hangry	1 2 3 4 5
4 hours between meals	1 2 3 4 5	Confidence	1 2 3 4 5
Energy levels	1 2 3 4 5	Stress levels	1 2 3 4 5
Digestion/Bloating	1 2 3 4 5	Sleep	1 2 3 4 5

What went well this week? What am I proud of?

_____

_____

_____

What was a struggle?

_____

_____

_____

Changes I'll make for next week:

_____

_____

_____

PREVIEW UPCOMING WEEK

Micro habit of the week: _____

What's happening this week: _____

_____

_____

How to navigate any obstacles to habits: _____

_____

_____

REVIEW PREVIOUS WEEK

DATE:

Rate yourself from 1 (it was a struggle) to 5 (100% full success!).

Micro habit	1 2 3 4 5	Cravings / Feeling hangry	1 2 3 4 5
4 hours between meals	1 2 3 4 5	Confidence	1 2 3 4 5
Energy levels	1 2 3 4 5	Stress levels	1 2 3 4 5
Digestion/Bloating	1 2 3 4 5	Sleep	1 2 3 4 5

What went well this week? What am I proud of?

_____
_____
_____

What was a struggle?

_____
_____
_____

Changes I'll make for next week:

_____
_____
_____
_____

PREVIEW UPCOMING WEEK

Micro habit of the week: _____

What's happening this week: _____

_____
_____
_____

How to navigate any obstacles to habits: _____

_____
_____
_____
_____

REVIEW PREVIOUS WEEK

DATE:

Rate yourself from 1 (it was a struggle) to 5 (100% full success!).

Micro habit	1 2 3 4 5	Cravings / Feeling hangry	1 2 3 4 5
4 hours between meals	1 2 3 4 5	Confidence	1 2 3 4 5
Energy levels	1 2 3 4 5	Stress levels	1 2 3 4 5
Digestion/Bloating	1 2 3 4 5	Sleep	1 2 3 4 5

What went well this week? What am I proud of?

What was a struggle?

Changes I'll make for next week:

PREVIEW UPCOMING WEEK

Micro habit of the week:

What's happening this week:

How to navigate any obstacles to habits:

REVIEW PREVIOUS WEEK

DATE:

Rate yourself from 1 (it was a struggle) to 5 (100% full success!).

Micro habit	1 2 3 4 5	Cravings / Feeling hangry	1 2 3 4 5
4 hours between meals	1 2 3 4 5	Confidence	1 2 3 4 5
Energy levels	1 2 3 4 5	Stress levels	1 2 3 4 5
Digestion/Bloating	1 2 3 4 5	Sleep	1 2 3 4 5

What went well this week? What am I proud of? _____

_____

_____

What was a struggle? _____

_____

_____

Changes I'll make for next week: _____

_____

_____

_____

PREVIEW UPCOMING WEEK

Micro habit of the week: _____

What's happening this week: _____

_____

_____

_____

How to navigate any obstacles to habits: _____

_____

_____

_____

REVIEW PREVIOUS WEEK

DATE:

Rate yourself from 1 (it was a struggle) to 5 (100% full success!).

Micro habit	1 2 3 4 5	Cravings / Feeling hangry	1 2 3 4 5
4 hours between meals	1 2 3 4 5	Confidence	1 2 3 4 5
Energy levels	1 2 3 4 5	Stress levels	1 2 3 4 5
Digestion/Bloating	1 2 3 4 5	Sleep	1 2 3 4 5

What went well this week? What am I proud of?

What was a struggle?

Changes I'll make for next week:

PREVIEW UPCOMING WEEK

Micro habit of the week:

What's happening this week:

How to navigate any obstacles to habits:

REVIEW PREVIOUS WEEK

DATE:

Rate yourself from 1 (it was a struggle) to 5 (100% full success!).

Micro habit	1 2 3 4 5	Cravings / Feeling hangry	1 2 3 4 5
4 hours between meals	1 2 3 4 5	Confidence	1 2 3 4 5
Energy levels	1 2 3 4 5	Stress levels	1 2 3 4 5
Digestion/Bloating	1 2 3 4 5	Sleep	1 2 3 4 5

What went well this week? What am I proud of?

_____

_____

What was a struggle?

_____

_____

Changes I'll make for next week:

_____

_____

_____

PREVIEW UPCOMING WEEK

Micro habit of the week: _____

What's happening this week: _____

_____

_____

How to navigate any obstacles to habits: _____

_____

_____

_____

REVIEW PREVIOUS WEEK

DATE:

Rate yourself from 1 (it was a struggle) to 5 (100% full success!).

Micro habit	1 2 3 4 5	Cravings / Feeling hangry	1 2 3 4 5
4 hours between meals	1 2 3 4 5	Confidence	1 2 3 4 5
Energy levels	1 2 3 4 5	Stress levels	1 2 3 4 5
Digestion/Bloating	1 2 3 4 5	Sleep	1 2 3 4 5

What went well this week? What am I proud of?

_____

_____

_____

What was a struggle?

_____

_____

_____

Changes I'll make for next week:

_____

_____

_____

_____

PREVIEW UPCOMING WEEK

Micro habit of the week: _____

What's happening this week: _____

_____

_____

_____

How to navigate any obstacles to habits: _____

_____

_____

_____

_____

REVIEW PREVIOUS WEEK

DATE:

Rate yourself from 1 (it was a struggle) to 5 (100% full success!).

Micro habit	1 2 3 4 5	Cravings / Feeling hangry	1 2 3 4 5
4 hours between meals	1 2 3 4 5	Confidence	1 2 3 4 5
Energy levels	1 2 3 4 5	Stress levels	1 2 3 4 5
Digestion/Bloating	1 2 3 4 5	Sleep	1 2 3 4 5

What went well this week? What am I proud of?

_____

_____

_____

What was a struggle?

_____

_____

_____

Changes I'll make for next week:

_____

_____

_____

PREVIEW UPCOMING WEEK

Micro habit of the week: _____

What's happening this week: _____

_____

_____

How to navigate any obstacles to habits: _____

_____

_____

_____

REVIEW PREVIOUS WEEK

DATE:

Rate yourself from 1 (it was a struggle) to 5 (100% full success!).

Micro habit	1 2 3 4 5	Cravings / Feeling hangry	1 2 3 4 5
4 hours between meals	1 2 3 4 5	Confidence	1 2 3 4 5
Energy levels	1 2 3 4 5	Stress levels	1 2 3 4 5
Digestion/Bloating	1 2 3 4 5	Sleep	1 2 3 4 5

What went well this week? What am I proud of?

What was a struggle?

Changes I'll make for next week:

PREVIEW UPCOMING WEEK

Micro habit of the week:

What's happening this week:

How to navigate any obstacles to habits:

REVIEW PREVIOUS WEEK

DATE:

Rate yourself from 1 (it was a struggle) to 5 (100% full success!).

Micro habit	1 2 3 4 5	Cravings / Feeling hangry	1 2 3 4 5
4 hours between meals	1 2 3 4 5	Confidence	1 2 3 4 5
Energy levels	1 2 3 4 5	Stress levels	1 2 3 4 5
Digestion/Bloating	1 2 3 4 5	Sleep	1 2 3 4 5

What went well this week? What am I proud of? _____
_____
_____

What was a struggle? _____
_____
_____

Changes I'll make for next week: _____
_____
_____
_____

PREVIEW UPCOMING WEEK

Micro habit of the week: _____

What's happening this week: _____
_____
_____
_____

How to navigate any obstacles to habits: _____
_____
_____
_____
_____

REVIEW PREVIOUS WEEK

DATE:

Rate yourself from 1 (it was a struggle) to 5 (100% full success!).

Micro habit	1 2 3 4 5	Cravings / Feeling hangry	1 2 3 4 5
4 hours between meals	1 2 3 4 5	Confidence	1 2 3 4 5
Energy levels	1 2 3 4 5	Stress levels	1 2 3 4 5
Digestion/Bloating	1 2 3 4 5	Sleep	1 2 3 4 5

What went well this week? What am I proud of?

What was a struggle?

Changes I'll make for next week:

PREVIEW UPCOMING WEEK

Micro habit of the week:

What's happening this week:

How to navigate any obstacles to habits:

REVIEW PREVIOUS WEEK

DATE:

Rate yourself from 1 (it was a struggle) to 5 (100% full success!).

Micro habit	1 2 3 4 5	Cravings / Feeling hangry	1 2 3 4 5
4 hours between meals	1 2 3 4 5	Confidence	1 2 3 4 5
Energy levels	1 2 3 4 5	Stress levels	1 2 3 4 5
Digestion/Bloating	1 2 3 4 5	Sleep	1 2 3 4 5

What went well this week? What am I proud of?

_____

_____

What was a struggle?

_____

_____

Changes I'll make for next week:

_____

_____

_____

PREVIEW UPCOMING WEEK

Micro habit of the week: _____

What's happening this week: _____

_____

_____

How to navigate any obstacles to habits: _____

_____

_____

_____

REVIEW PREVIOUS WEEK

DATE:

Rate yourself from 1 (it was a struggle) to 5 (100% full success!).

Micro habit	1 2 3 4 5	Cravings / Feeling hangry	1 2 3 4 5
4 hours between meals	1 2 3 4 5	Confidence	1 2 3 4 5
Energy levels	1 2 3 4 5	Stress levels	1 2 3 4 5
Digestion/Bloating	1 2 3 4 5	Sleep	1 2 3 4 5

What went well this week? What am I proud of?

What was a struggle?

Changes I'll make for next week:

PREVIEW UPCOMING WEEK

Micro habit of the week:

What's happening this week:

How to navigate any obstacles to habits:

REVIEW PREVIOUS WEEK

DATE:

Rate yourself from 1 (it was a struggle) to 5 (100% full success!).

Micro habit	1 2 3 4 5	Cravings / Feeling hangry	1 2 3 4 5
4 hours between meals	1 2 3 4 5	Confidence	1 2 3 4 5
Energy levels	1 2 3 4 5	Stress levels	1 2 3 4 5
Digestion/Bloating	1 2 3 4 5	Sleep	1 2 3 4 5

What went well this week? What am I proud of?

What was a struggle?

Changes I'll make for next week:

PREVIEW UPCOMING WEEK

Micro habit of the week:

What's happening this week:

How to navigate any obstacles to habits:

REVIEW PREVIOUS WEEK

DATE:

Rate yourself from 1 (it was a struggle) to 5 (100% full success!).

Micro habit	1 2 3 4 5	Cravings / Feeling hangry	1 2 3 4 5
4 hours between meals	1 2 3 4 5	Confidence	1 2 3 4 5
Energy levels	1 2 3 4 5	Stress levels	1 2 3 4 5
Digestion/Bloating	1 2 3 4 5	Sleep	1 2 3 4 5

What went well this week? What am I proud of?

_____

_____

What was a struggle?

_____

_____

Changes I'll make for next week:

_____

_____

PREVIEW UPCOMING WEEK

Micro habit of the week: _____

What's happening this week: _____

_____

_____

How to navigate any obstacles to habits: _____

_____

_____

_____

REVIEW PREVIOUS WEEK

DATE:

Rate yourself from 1 (it was a struggle) to 5 (100% full success!).

Micro habit	1 2 3 4 5	Cravings / Feeling hangry	1 2 3 4 5
4 hours between meals	1 2 3 4 5	Confidence	1 2 3 4 5
Energy levels	1 2 3 4 5	Stress levels	1 2 3 4 5
Digestion/Bloating	1 2 3 4 5	Sleep	1 2 3 4 5

What went well this week? What am I proud of?

What was a struggle?

Changes I'll make for next week:

PREVIEW UPCOMING WEEK

Micro habit of the week:

What's happening this week:

How to navigate any obstacles to habits:

REVIEW PREVIOUS WEEK

DATE:

Rate yourself from 1 (it was a struggle) to 5 (100% full success!).

Micro habit	1 2 3 4 5	Cravings / Feeling hangry	1 2 3 4 5
4 hours between meals	1 2 3 4 5	Confidence	1 2 3 4 5
Energy levels	1 2 3 4 5	Stress levels	1 2 3 4 5
Digestion/Bloating	1 2 3 4 5	Sleep	1 2 3 4 5

What went well this week? What am I proud of?

What was a struggle?

Changes I'll make for next week:

PREVIEW UPCOMING WEEK

Micro habit of the week:

What's happening this week:

How to navigate any obstacles to habits:

REVIEW PREVIOUS WEEK

DATE:

Rate yourself from 1 (it was a struggle) to 5 (100% full success!).

Micro habit	1 2 3 4 5	Cravings / Feeling hangry	1 2 3 4 5
4 hours between meals	1 2 3 4 5	Confidence	1 2 3 4 5
Energy levels	1 2 3 4 5	Stress levels	1 2 3 4 5
Digestion/Bloating	1 2 3 4 5	Sleep	1 2 3 4 5

What went well this week? What am I proud of?

_____
_____

What was a struggle?

_____
_____

Changes I'll make for next week:

_____
_____
_____

PREVIEW UPCOMING WEEK

Micro habit of the week: _____

What's happening this week: _____

_____
_____
_____

How to navigate any obstacles to habits: _____

_____
_____
_____

REVIEW PREVIOUS WEEK

DATE:

Rate yourself from 1 (it was a struggle) to 5 (100% full success!).

Micro habit	1 2 3 4 5	Cravings / Feeling hangry 1 2 3 4 5
4 hours between meals	1 2 3 4 5	Confidence 1 2 3 4 5
Energy levels	1 2 3 4 5	Stress levels 1 2 3 4 5
Digestion/Bloating	1 2 3 4 5	Sleep 1 2 3 4 5

What went well this week? What am I proud of?

What was a struggle?

Changes I'll make for next week:

PREVIEW UPCOMING WEEK

Micro habit of the week:

What's happening this week:

How to navigate any obstacles to habits:

REVIEW PREVIOUS WEEK

DATE:

Rate yourself from 1 (it was a struggle) to 5 (100% full success!).

Micro habit	1 2 3 4 5	Cravings / Feeling hangry	1 2 3 4 5
4 hours between meals	1 2 3 4 5	Confidence	1 2 3 4 5
Energy levels	1 2 3 4 5	Stress levels	1 2 3 4 5
Digestion/Bloating	1 2 3 4 5	Sleep	1 2 3 4 5

What went well this week? What am I proud of?

_____

_____

What was a struggle?

_____

_____

Changes I'll make for next week:

_____

_____

_____

PREVIEW UPCOMING WEEK

Micro habit of the week: _____

What's happening this week: _____

_____

_____

How to navigate any obstacles to habits: _____

_____

_____

_____

REVIEW PREVIOUS WEEK

DATE:

Rate yourself from 1 (it was a struggle) to 5 (100% full success!).

Micro habit	1 2 3 4 5	Cravings / Feeling hangry	1 2 3 4 5
4 hours between meals	1 2 3 4 5	Confidence	1 2 3 4 5
Energy levels	1 2 3 4 5	Stress levels	1 2 3 4 5
Digestion/Bloating	1 2 3 4 5	Sleep	1 2 3 4 5

What went well this week? What am I proud of?

_____

_____

What was a struggle?

_____

_____

Changes I'll make for next week:

_____

_____

_____

PREVIEW UPCOMING WEEK

Micro habit of the week: _____

What's happening this week: _____

_____

_____

How to navigate any obstacles to habits: _____

_____

_____

_____

REVIEW PREVIOUS WEEK

DATE:

Rate yourself from 1 (it was a struggle) to 5 (100% full success!).

Micro habit	1 2 3 4 5	Cravings / Feeling hangry	1 2 3 4 5
4 hours between meals	1 2 3 4 5	Confidence	1 2 3 4 5
Energy levels	1 2 3 4 5	Stress levels	1 2 3 4 5
Digestion/Bloating	1 2 3 4 5	Sleep	1 2 3 4 5

What went well this week? What am I proud of?

_____

_____

What was a struggle?

_____

_____

Changes I'll make for next week:

_____

_____

_____

PREVIEW UPCOMING WEEK

Micro habit of the week: _____

What's happening this week: _____

_____

_____

How to navigate any obstacles to habits: _____

_____

_____

_____

REVIEW PREVIOUS WEEK

DATE:

Rate yourself from 1 (it was a struggle) to 5 (100% full success!).

Micro habit	1 2 3 4 5	Cravings / Feeling hangry 1 2 3 4 5
4 hours between meals	1 2 3 4 5	Confidence 1 2 3 4 5
Energy levels	1 2 3 4 5	Stress levels 1 2 3 4 5
Digestion/Bloating	1 2 3 4 5	Sleep 1 2 3 4 5

What went well this week? What am I proud of?

_____

_____

What was a struggle?

_____

_____

Changes I'll make for next week:

_____

_____

_____

PREVIEW UPCOMING WEEK

Micro habit of the week: _____

What's happening this week: _____

_____

_____

How to navigate any obstacles to habits: _____

_____

_____

_____

REVIEW PREVIOUS WEEK

DATE:

Rate yourself from 1 (it was a struggle) to 5 (100% full success!).

Micro habit	1 2 3 4 5	Cravings / Feeling hangry	1 2 3 4 5
4 hours between meals	1 2 3 4 5	Confidence	1 2 3 4 5
Energy levels	1 2 3 4 5	Stress levels	1 2 3 4 5
Digestion/Bloating	1 2 3 4 5	Sleep	1 2 3 4 5

What went well this week? What am I proud of?

_____

_____

_____

What was a struggle?

_____

_____

_____

Changes I'll make for next week:

_____

_____

_____

PREVIEW UPCOMING WEEK

Micro habit of the week: _____

What's happening this week: _____

_____

_____

_____

How to navigate any obstacles to habits: _____

_____

_____

_____

REVIEW PREVIOUS WEEK

DATE:

Rate yourself from 1 (it was a struggle) to 5 (100% full success!).

Micro habit	1 2 3 4 5	Cravings / Feeling hangry	1 2 3 4 5
4 hours between meals	1 2 3 4 5	Confidence	1 2 3 4 5
Energy levels	1 2 3 4 5	Stress levels	1 2 3 4 5
Digestion/Bloating	1 2 3 4 5	Sleep	1 2 3 4 5

What went well this week? What am I proud of?

_____

_____

What was a struggle?

_____

_____

Changes I'll make for next week:

_____

_____

PREVIEW UPCOMING WEEK

Micro habit of the week: _____

What's happening this week: _____

_____

_____

How to navigate any obstacles to habits: _____

_____

_____

_____

Rate yourself from 1 (it was a struggle) to 5 (100% full success!).

Micro habit	1 2 3 4 5	Cravings / Feeling hangry	1 2 3 4 5
4 hours between meals	1 2 3 4 5	Confidence	1 2 3 4 5
Energy levels	1 2 3 4 5	Stress levels	1 2 3 4 5
Digestion/Bloating	1 2 3 4 5	Sleep	1 2 3 4 5

What went well this week? What am I proud of? _____

_____

_____

What was a struggle? _____

_____

_____

Changes I'll make for next week: _____

_____

_____

You did it! *I'm so proud that you have completed a full year of making over your metabolism! I hope you continue to grow and evolve into the version of YOU that you know exists, and that you remember your body is not a project—committing to yourself does not have an end date. I have been using the methods in this book for five years, and my body, health, and life are always improving through the growth I experience using the same pages you just completed.*

Love,
Megan

RESOURCES

To make life easier for you, I've created a resource section! Here you'll find a short list of good places to get information, products, tools, and other resources to help you this year. This list is constantly growing and evolving, so if you'd like more up-to-date suggestions, please go to the Metabolism Makeover website (metabolismmakeover.co/resources), and I will keep you in the loop.

PHFF ESSENTIALS: WHAT'S ALWAYS IN MY KITCHEN

Here is a peek inside my kitchen! I create "throw together" meals, matching a protein, a healthy fat, fiber, and starchy carbs more than I make actual recipes, because I find it to be quicker and easier for meal prep. My staples remain pretty steady, and I wanted to give you some of my favorite, Megan-approved brands to look out for. Typically, I'll make a couple of proteins, vegetables, and starchy carbs at the beginning of the week and combine as I go, adding fat to each meal.

You absolutely do not have to buy organic, free-range, pastured anything. This is my personal preference, but I want you to focus only on doing what you can to have steady blood sugars when you eat. To build this list, I went into my fully stocked kitchen and made notes on what I had on hand and brand names.

Proteins

I love shopping at Costco for organic (or not!) proteins. Buy these in bulk to save lots of cash!

- ☐ chicken nuggets (Just Bare)
- ☐ cottage cheese (Good Culture)
- ☐ Greek yogurt (Fage or Siggi's)
- ☐ organic chicken breasts, chicken thighs, ground beef, and wild shrimp (Costco)
- ☐ eggs from pastured chickens (local farm)
- ☐ protein powders: Just Ingredients (for plant-based powders, I recommend Truvani, and for egg-based ones, Designer Wellness)
- ☐ protein bars: Aloha (I also recommend Paleovalley, Nash Bars, and RXBARs)

Healthy Fats

- ☐ avocados
- ☐ cashews, pistachios, Brazil nuts (Thrive Market)
- ☐ cashew butter (Georgia Grinders)
- ☐ cheese (I mix it up!)
- ☐ coconut milk (Native Forest)
- ☐ guacamole cups (Costco)
- ☐ hummus cups (Costco)
- ☐ peanut butter (Georgia Grinders)

Fiber

- ☐ chia seeds (Thrive Market)
- ☐ frozen organic berries (Costco)
- ☐ frozen organic vegetables (Costco)
- ☐ microgreens
- ☐ prepped raw or cooked vegetables like broccoli, cauliflower, cucumbers, and carrots
- ☐ salad greens
- ☐ variety of fresh fruits

Starchy Carbs

- ☐ avocado-oil potato chips (Siete or Thrive Market)
- ☐ beans (any kind)
- ☐ crackers (Simple Mills)
- ☐ grain-free tortilla chips (Siete or Thrive Market)
- ☐ jasmine rice (Lundberg)
- ☐ lentils (Tasty Bite)
- ☐ potatoes (we do a variety!)
- ☐ flour tortillas

Condiments

- ☐ coconut aminos (Bragg)
- ☐ mustard, Dijon and yellow
- ☐ pickles (Bubbies)
- ☐ salsa (any kind without added sugar)

Treats

- ☐ full-fat ice cream (Alden's)
- ☐ popsicles (JonnyPops)

Alcohol

I'm not a big drinker, but if I do drink, this is what I pick up.

- ☐ Dry Farm Wines
- ☐ Scout & Cellar
- ☐ unflavored vodka, gin, tequila, rum, or whiskey with no added sugar
- ☐ club soda, mineral water, or seltzers like Poppi or OLIPOP
- ☐ fresh fruit, cucumber slices, and herbs for garnish
- ☐ lemons and limes

PHFF RECIPES

Find my favorite PHFF recipes at metabolismmakeover.co/resources.

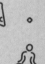

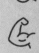
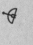
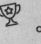

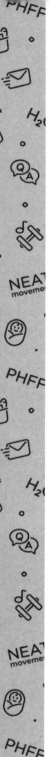

WORKOUTS

On page 8, you found a three-day strength-training program; at metabolismmakeover .co/resources, you will find the videos that go along with this program, plus a no-equipment program for beginners, travel days, or those days you just need to squeeze something in on your living room floor. If you'll be doing your strength training at home, you will need:

- two to three sets of dumbbells or resistance bands (keep in mind, as you progress, you'll need to gradually go up in weight)
- a bench

There is no need to buy fancy equipment. You can often find dumbbells at consignment stores or secondhand online for a great price. Fabric dumbbells (rather than metal) tend to be the most comfortable to hold. As for a bench, you may be able to find something around the house, like an ottoman or decorative bench (just make sure it's sturdy!).

Other recommended progressive overload strength programs: Mind Pump Media, Paragon Training Methods, Moves by Madeline, and Sohee Fit.

TOOLS

There are so many cool biohacking tools on the market, but many of them can be pricey. My advice is to start small, and once you've done the foundational free stuff (PHFF! morning light! meditation!) and you begin to see improvements, add another tool or two to optimize. Or don't!

RISE App (risescience.com)
This app helps track your sleep debt, and it is wonderful for holding you accountable on sleep. You'll notice that as sleep debt increases, energy decreases. I personally work hard to keep sleep debt under 10 hours (in a two-week cycle), because I know that once I hit 10 hours, my energy levels really tank.

Bon Charge Blue Light Blocking Glasses (boncharge.com)
There are plenty of blue-light blockers on the market, but I like Bon Charge's because they are high quality *and* stylish. Make sure your blue-light blockers have been tested for effectiveness and that they have a red tint (which is what blocks out blue light at night).

Oura Ring (ouraring.com)
While Oura is most known for tracking sleep, it also collects data on over 20 biometrics that directly impact your health and well-being. It takes this data and gives you targeted recommendations.

Signos Continuous Blood Glucose Monitor (signos.com)
This continuous glucose monitor (CGM) sends your blood sugar data via Bluetooth to the Signos app, where you can track your blood sugar levels and see how your body responds to the food you eat.

Truvaga (truvaga.com)
This device gently activates your vagus nerve, helping your body manage its fight-or-flight response with just a two-minute session twice per day.

SUPPLEMENT BRANDS

Targeted supplementation can be a game changer for many, but the supplement industry is the Wild West; choosing pure, high-quality supplements is necessary, unless you want to flush your money down the toilet (literally—if you're taking supplements your body can't even absorb, you'll be flushing them down the toilet). The supplements listed here are my absolute favorite, trusted brands:

- *Epsoak Epsom Salt:* Not only does heat in the form of a bath, shower, or sauna in the evening help you sleep by lowering your core body temperature, but adding muscle-relaxing magnesium sulfate to your bath can also help your body and mind actually relax before bedtime.
- *Just Thrive:* This is one of the few probiotics clinically proven to "arrive alive" in the gut, where it belongs.
- *Garden of Life Organic Vegan Sport Protein Powder:* This high-quality plant-based protein powder has a full amino acid profile in the appropriate amounts to trigger muscle protein synthesis.
- *Kion Aminos Capsules:* This amino supplement includes all nine essential amino acids, which helps support building lean muscle and muscle recovery.
- *Just Ingredients Protein Powder:* This whole-food protein powder is flavored with real ingredients.

- *Urban Moonshine Digestive Bitters:* I prefer a liquid product, and while the taste isn't so great, adding your bitters to a small spray bottle and spraying it into your mouth before meals can help with the taste.

Mineral Brand Options

- *Jigsaw:* This electrolyte powder comes with bioavailable vitamins and minerals.
- *Just Ingredients:* This electrolyte powder is made primarily with whole-food ingredients.
- *LMNT:* If you're doing sweaty workouts, sauna, coffee enemas, or anything that is particularly dehydrating, LMNT is a high-sodium electrolyte product that will help replace what you lose through sweat.
- *Rayvi:* This is a high-quality, high-potassium electrolyte powder.
- *Re-Lyte:* This is another tasty electrolyte powder with bioavailable vitamins and minerals.

Lab Tests

- *Hair tissue mineral analysis (HTMA):* The HTMA measures the levels of minerals and heavy metals found in hair. This test has become one of my favorites as it offers an affordable insight into gut health, thyroid function, adrenal health, inflammation, heavy metal toxicity, mineral imbalances, immune function, and more. Starting with an HTMA can prevent you from spending money on expensive tests you may not need. To order a test kit and receive a personalized plan from one of our HTMA-trained functional dietitians, go to metabolismmakeover.co/htma.
- *GI-MAP, a.k.a. a gut test:* Getting a gut health test is an excellent window into your digestive health that can help uncover the root cause of your digestive or skin issues. It takes a look at the balance of good and bad bacteria, parasites, pathogens, and viruses. It also can provide insights into your immune system, how well you are absorbing the nutrients you are consuming, and inflammation levels. To work with one of our dietitians specializing in gut health, go to metabolismmakeover.co/vip.

ACKNOWLEDGMENTS

This workbook organizes all of the exercises that I have created, tested, and used with clients who have lost up to 100+ lbs—and kept it off—over the years. Women healing their bodies and their relationship with food goes far beyond themselves—it changes generations to come. I am honored to walk next to all of you who are making the decision to commit to YOU.

To Elizabeth, my publishing coach, who supported me in bringing my vision to life after a dozen iterations of this project (literally).

To Jess, who came up with the concept of YOU. It couldn't describe the women using this workbook any better.

To Cierra and Helena, who always pick up the slack when I decide to go off the grid and write another book I swore I wasn't going to write.

I want to thank my hybrid publisher, Flashpoint, who wholeheartedly supports my vision of this work.

And finally, the Metabolism Makeover community, who took a chance and believed me when I said changing their bodies started in their minds, and not on their plates.

ABOUT THE AUTHOR

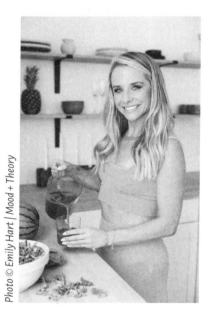

Megan Hansen, a registered dietitian nutritionist, is the founder and CEO of Metabolism Makeover—a virtual nutrition-coaching business with a focus on weight loss and metabolic health. With a community of almost 40 dietitians and over eight thousand past and present clients, Hansen's company is dedicated to helping clients learn how to change their relationship with food so that they can lose the weight—and the food anxiety— and keep it off for good. As a speaker and industry leader, Hansen has been featured in *EatingWell*, *Martha Stewart Living* magazine, and the *Skinny Confidential*. She lives in Atlanta, Georgia. Visit her website at www.metabolismmakeover.co.